THE AFRICAN-AMERICAN GUIDE TO
HEPATITIS C

SAMUEL J. DANIEL, M.D., F.A.C.P., F.A.C.G.

TEMIMA MARKOVITS, R.P.A.-C.
VERNON A. WILLIAMS

HILTON PUBLISHING COMPANY · CHICAGO, ILLINOIS

Hilton Publishing Company
Chicago, IL

Direct all correspondence to:
Hilton Publishing Company
110 Ridge Road
Munster, IN 46321
815-885-1070
www.hiltonpub.com

The information and opinions contained in this book may not necessarily be those of Roche or the publisher.

Notice: The information in this book is true and complete to the best knowledge of the authors, publisher, and Roche. This book is intended only as an information reference and should not replace, countermand, or conflict with the advice given to readers by their physicians. The authors, publisher, and Roche disclaim all liability in connection with the specific personal use of any and all information provided in this book.

Library of Congress Cataloging-in-Publication Data

Daniel, Samuel J.
    The African-American Guide to Hepatitis C / by Samuel J. Daniel, Temima Markovits, Vernon A. Williams.
        p. cm.
    Includes bibliographical references and index.
    ISBN 0-9716067-2-2 (pbk. : alk. paper)
    1. Hepatitis C—popular works. 2. African Americans—Diseases—Popular works. I. Markovits, Temima. II. Williams, Vernon A. III. Title.
    RC848.H425D36 2005
    616.3'623—dc22   2005000831

Printed and bound in the United States of America

CONTENTS

ACKNOWLEDGMENTS

We would like to acknowledge all our past and present patients afflicted with chronic Hepatitis C. Without you this book could not have been written. You inspired it. As our institution has been addressing this serious health problem in recent years, we have come to understand your needs as individuals, as well as your needs as members of an African-American community. By your questions, your comments, your praises, and your criticism, we have been able to fine-tune our approach to the management of your disease. Just as spouses in a good marriage teach one another how to nurture and love, you have taught us and guided us on how to take care of you, how to escort you through your treatment, how to share your successes and disappointments.

Each one of you is unique and has unique needs, yet you also share common issues with others afflicted with the same disease. Recognizing the needs of an African-

American community significantly affected by Hepatitis C has further inspired us to lay the foundation for the formation of our future center of excellence for the treatment of hepatitis.

We also have to thank every member of our hospital staff—all our tireless physicians, radiology staff, nurses, clinical assistants, laboratory personnel, administrators, secretaries, clerks, and housekeeping staff. Each one of you has played an important role in this teamwork. Each one of you has helped develop our unique structure that fosters patient satisfaction by ensuring our patients are welcomed in a respectful, friendly, and professional manner in an institution that takes pride in maintaining a high standard of cleanliness and aesthetics.

Finally, we have to thank the pharmaceutical companies for their efforts in researching and developing medications that are now standard of care and that offer increased hope of overcoming Hepatitis C. We also thank them for their various programs that address the needs of the underserved communities. These pharmaceutical companies have further contributed by instituting drug reimbursement assistance programs for patients without insurance and by providing educational activities to help clinicians, at all levels, keep abreast of cutting-edge medical knowledge.

We also thank the various scientific associations, such as the American Association for the Study of Liver Diseases (AASLD), the American Gastroenterology Association (AGA), the American College of

Gastroenterology (ACG), as well as the United States government's Centers for Disease Control (CDC), for their contribution to the wealth of our knowledge base by holding international annual meetings, symposia and consensus conferences that gather experts from around the world who share the results of their investigations and continually keep us abreast of new findings and recommendations.

We are especially indebted to our families and loved ones, who have patiently supported us in our zeal to keep informed and cultivate various relationships in the academic community, by participating in the various scientific meetings all over the country where new research and new guidelines are constantly being developed. Those evenings and weekends away from home at these conferences allowed us to gain expertise in the field of managing chronic Hepatitis C by learning from all the international and national experts in liver disease.

Samuel J. Daniel, M.D.

INTRODUCTION

Killer Ray is one of the country's most respected jazz drummers. When he was fifteen, he trained under Wes Montgomery. Killer Ray has played with such music legends as John Coltrane and Freddie Hubbard. Like many top jazz musicians, Killer Ray happens to be African American.

Killer Ray's early years of fame meant hard work but it also meant parties, alcohol, and drugs. It was years later, in 1999, that a routine blood test revealed he had Hepatitis C. That was the beginning of a story that had many ups and downs. But Killer Ray, once he faced the facts, understood that he had to learn more about his disease in order to be able to work effectively with his doctors, in a partnership whose only business was his good health.

Killer Ray worked hard to learn what he needed to know even when it concerned the fact that he had the worst possible strain of the virus, called genotype 1. Ray learned and understood that this strain was hardest to treat. He faced this reality and did what he had to do. He enrolled in a clinical trial using a new medication and, through a process that went on for a year, was successfully treated. Two years later, Ray was still virus free. He understood that by being a part of a test he would be helping not just himself, but others whose lives might later be saved by the experimental medication he was taking. In fact, that is how it turned out. As a result of the clinical trial Killer Ray and others were part of, the Food and Drug Administration (FDA) has now approved the medication they tested.

Today, Killer Ray is, gratefully, back on stage drumming with newfound energy. But he never forgets that he was one of the lucky ones. There are lots of men out in the communities who need to learn what he did about the importance of getting diagnosed at the early stages of Hepatitis C, when it can be treated most effectively. Ray also learned that the disease is more prevalent among African Americans than any other racial group.

Killer Ray is a deeply spiritual person, a practicing Buddhist. So his heart is tuned to gratitude for his own blessings and, at the same time, tuned to love of others. He gave life to that love by his vow to spread the knowledge about this disease that has the frightening nickname of "silent killer," which is what Hepatitis C can be if it is not diagnosed and treated. Ray's message to anyone who may have been exposed to the disease is simple and direct: *"Get informed, get evaluated, do not bury your head in the ground and make believe you are not sick. Find a doctor you trust who knows about the disease, and, if he judges that you could benefit from treatment, get treated."*

Once Killer Ray accepted the hard fact that he had Hepatitis C, he practiced the same message he would later preach. Ray trusted his doctor's ability to present the facts and then, in discussion with Ray, review treatment options with him. Ray was able to hold up his end of the discussion because he knew the facts about his disease. Ray trusted the decision they had agreed upon. He trusted it even though he knew it meant he would be taking a treatment that sometimes had severe side effects, a treatment that came with no guarantees.

During his treatment for Hepatitis C, Ray formed a close bond with his doctors, his physician assistant, the research director at the hospital, the secretaries, and the clerks. Ray was in an environment he already trusted, where his other medical conditions had been stabilized, where his good leg had been saved, and where he knew he was loved and cared for. Ray was also in a unique environment where most of the staff in the hospital he was in were African American—from the president and the administrators, to the doctors, nurses, clerks, cooks, housekeeping staff, and engineering staff.

Ray found himself surrounded by competent, capable people in a cultural atmosphere that was completely familiar to him, and where his own charm and smile just reflected those of his environment. He recognized that if there was to be any chance of successful treatment, there had to be teamwork, and that team included him as the most important player.

Killer Ray chanted his way through treatment, and he continues to chant—for the end of all human suffering and for the cure of all illnesses.

KILLER RAY TELLS HIS STORY

When I first found out I had Hepatitis C, in 1999, I did not want to deal with it! At the time, I had just found out that I had diabetes and that I was probably going to lose my right leg, so I had enough headaches—without Hepatitis! I had been drug free for a few years and had stopped drinking booze. I was struggling to get my act together. On top of all that, I am now asked to deal with some stupid virus they said I probably got when I was drugging and drinking. Anyway, I was clean, and I did not want to be reminded of the bad old days. Those years were finally gone, and I was willing to deal with my diabetes and try to save my leg. I did not care about my liver. To tell you the honest truth, I did not even know where my liver was.

So I just put off the hepatitis thing, though I was not exactly taking a holiday. I started insulin treatment for the diabetes. I had a fem-pop on my right leg. [Fem-pop is medical jargon that stands for a femoral-popliteal bypass surgery.] The bypass operation meant taking a vein from my good leg and grafting it in my bad leg to try to save it. The bad leg had poor circulation because of years of having diabetes and not knowing that I had it. I was a musician too busy jamming and drugging and partying and totally unconcerned about my health—until I landed in an emergency room with gangrene setting in my toes!

For me, becoming healthy meant getting my blood pressure, as well as my diabetes, under control. (The doctors called my high blood pressure "hypertension.") I understood that these two conditions were so often found together in the African-American community that you might call them part of our African heritage.

Because I was going through all that medical stuff, it is not surprising that I was still in denial about the Hepatitis C. I returned to the clinic, where I learned that my liver enzymes were abnormal. Enzymes? Chemicals in my liver that increase with inflammation! I had just gone through an amputation, and the pain was finally under control. I was adjusting to being handicapped, so now, though I took in the new bad news about the Hepatitis C, my heart still resisted.

So I kept on arguing. "I do not feel sick," I told my doctors. "I just feel hungry, and I can not eat as much bread as I want because it is filled with too many carbohydrates!" I was really getting smart with medical words. By now I knew that carbohydrates are found in sugar, bread, rice, macaroni salad— all the good things! My diet was like a conspiracy that kept me from eating anything good.

My doctor patiently let me know that my problem was more serious than hunger. Even after I accepted the fact, I kept arguing for a while. The whole thing seemed unfair, even cruel. Why me? I am not the only one who played around! Why are some people lucky and not me? I already had my share of troubles. My life was getting better. I was learning how to use my plastic leg—what the doctors called a prosthesis.

But I got over the self-pity, too. I had chanted, as a Buddhist, to give me strength and direction while I went through my earlier ordeals. I used chants again now. Then I was ready to ask a lot of questions, and take in the answers. But when the doctor started to tell me about biopsy and treatment options, I just refused to hear. All I agreed to is that I would come back again for my next appointment.

During the follow-up appointment, the doctors I talked to did not push me to undergo treatment. But they did give me a lot of information. I trusted them. The rest was up to me. The doctors offered me the option of a biopsy, and of being included in a clinical trial that was testing a new form of interferon. The decision whether or not to accept their offer was entirely mine.

I had already learned what happened when you did not deal with diabetes: I lost my leg. I also knew that if I did not carefully manage my hypertension, I would probably have a heart attack. And that can kill you with no warning! I felt like a walking time bomb.

But I had taken care of myself and managed both of these diseases. I was doing pretty good. My kidneys were working, and my eye doctor told me that so far I was lucky. My heart was beating normally, and my blood pressure was almost normal. I had a good doctor who told me that "almost" is not good enough, so I was on three or four different pills to bring the pressure down to normal! To my surprise, I'd become a good patient.

Facing the treatment option, I thought to myself: "Now that my heart and diabetes are improving, what if my liver disease kills me?" So, reluctantly, back at the clinic, I let my negative energy disappear. The "doctor" I talked to was actually a physician assistant [PA], trained to diagnose and treat patients, and to assist the doctors in other ways as well. The PA carefully *explained the disease to me, and let me know that Hepatitis C could cause cirrhosis. If I had cirrhosis, I could get liver cancer or my liver could stop working and I would need a transplant. The PA explained that a biopsy was the only way to find out how much damage had been done to my liver because of Hepatitis C and because of my boozing. I was at risk. The doctors said I was a "double hitter"! My liver was "hit" twice: by alcohol and by a virus—double damage!*

The possibility of cancer and a transplant scared me. The doctors told me the truth. Not everybody gets cirrhosis, only about 20 percent of those who have Hepatitis C. And not everybody that has cirrhosis gets cancer: only 5 percent. Still as Hepatitis C progressed, there was a serious chance that one day I would need a transplant. Would I take a chance now to prevent that? The new treatment they recommended had around a 50 percent chance of success.

I chanted and I chanted and asked more questions. The doctors explained to me that the biopsy they wanted to take—that is, the very small sample of my liver tissue that they would take with a needle—had a small risk of causing bleeding because the liver has a lot of blood vessels in it. Even with the risk, I agreed to have the biopsy. The reason I was willing to go ahead with it is that I trusted the doctors were telling me the truth. I also trusted that they really cared about me and wanted to work with me to try to cure me. I was Killer Ray, I was a fighter with my drums, I was a fighter who had fought hard to save my leg, I was going to fight again to get rid of the Hep C virus.

That was in May 2000. After that, I took treatment for 48 weeks—338 days. It was a long, sometimes difficult period. Getting through it took a lot of encouragement from others, patience on the part of my doctors, and courage on my own part. As a result of the treatment, I experienced bad symptoms. I had anemia. I suffered from fatigue. My hair thinned out. I was sweating.

I complained. I called on the phone. I was tired, yet sometimes I could not sleep. I chanted, I asked for help and said thank you. Sometimes I felt a little irritable and a little down, but I was encouraged by the early results of my week 12 viral load test: the Hepatitis C virus was not detectable! I appreciated the good news, to put it mildly, and my doctors were happy with me and for me. They were good to me, and the staff watched over me and gave me encouragement or special care when that is what I needed, along with occasional pokes to find veins where there weren't any. The reward for our work was that the initial results were good.

At six months of treatment, the virus was undetectable! That was music to my ears. The good news encouraged me more. I chanted and chanted, and took those injections and those pills. I wanted to help myself. Today, in August 2003, I look back. I have been virus free for 26 months.

I cannot get used to saying I do not have Hepatitis C. A lot of my fellow musicians are still struggling with it. Some of them started treatment but could not see it through. Treatment back then was an injection three times a week, not the new, stronger, longer-acting injection that is now taken only once a week. Some of my friends still have the virus, and others who should have gotten diagnosed had not. All I can tell them is that, though there are no guarantees, interferon treatment definitely helps the liver in many ways. Look at me! I can play the drums just like before.

I am playing my drums better now than ever before, and I am still chanting. Just as I chanted to help get myself through my ordeals, I keep on chanting—for continued success in my career, for world peace, and for the end of this serious disease.

WHY RAY'S STORY MATTERS AND WHY THIS BOOK AT THIS TIME?

We chose Ray's story as an introduction because it captures many of the feelings, fears, objections, and questions that people who have Hepatitis C have when they are first diagnosed with the disease, when they consider treatment, and when they go through treatment. This story also emphasizes how important it is for the patient to become an active partner in the process of healing. Such partnership is the first step to recovery.

The African-American community is not yet fully informed about Hepatitis C, and too many of our folks do not yet know they have the infection. How then can we help prevent complications of the disease if it is not even being diagnosed? As we remind you throughout this book, knowledge is power. Community centers, churches, temples, and mosques must help raise public awareness about Hepatitis C. Your primary-care physician should screen all patients who have had exposure to the risk factors of the disease and should hand out information about it. Where are the Hepatitis C walkathons? Hopefully, they are coming soon.

Among the first questions asked by those who have just been diagnosed are, "What is Hepatitis C?" "How did I get it?" and "What does it mean to my future health?" *The African-American Guide to Hepatitis C* is designed to set forth, in layman's terms, what Hepatitis C is and how it affects the body. This book also outlines lifestyle changes and precautions that can prevent the spread of the disease, and pays particular attention to the problems that face African Americans in the diagnosis, testing, and treatment of Hepatitis C. Finally, *The African-American Guide to Hepatitis C* explores treatment options and shows you how you can manage the disease if you get it. As you will soon learn, as an African American you are part of a group that is most at risk from this disease. By learning what you need to know, you will not only be helping to protect yourself, but you may also become involved with others in advocating wider understanding in the larger community, and advocating for more research for a vaccine and cure.

As you will see throughout this book, the dynamics between patient and caregiver are of primary importance. On the patient's part, it means being committed to seeking information, asking questions, and finding the physician and health center that offers the best care that meets his or her needs. On the part of the health care team—the doctor, physician assistant, nurse practitioner, nurse, medical assistant—commitment means delivering proper patient care in the most efficient and genuinely sympathetic way possible.

We are addressing you as an individual reader, and our first concern is your well-being. But as you know, no man is an island. We have brothers and sisters at large who have similar concerns and similar needs. When a community such as ours faces a serious health problem, we find strength in consolidating our efforts. We have found that we need to rally all our resources to be effective and defeat disease.

We have learned from HIV centers that it requires a lot of effort to manage the many aspects of a chronic illness. You can see in Ray's story that he relied on a number of different people for support. We have come to acknowledge our responsibility to your people in setting the foundation for a center that is going to address all the needs of those afflicted with Hepatitis C. We are facing the reality that this is not a single doctor–single patient relationship; there is a larger picture that takes into consideration all the needs of the patient as a whole.

Our community is full of brave "Killer Rays" who have turned their lives around but are still struggling with Hepatitis C. Minorities have everything to gain by uniting their strengths and forming centers of excellence to address the growing need for comprehensive care for any given illness. You can search the Internet and find numerous Web sites about centers of excellence for various illnesses and various racial groups. If you do not have a computer, you can go to the library and ask the librarian to help you. The resource section at the end of this book contains some suggestions for getting started in your search.

As a service to our own community, we have started to tap into various resources, rallying supporters to help us manage Hepatitis C as well as many other diseases that affect our brothers and sisters in a disproportionate fashion. We view our patients with affection and compassion as members of our greater family. Their trials and successes are ours as well. Within a center of excellence, there is improved communication between all the different disciplines, between medical clinicians, psychiatrists, social workers, and all others. As a member of your community, you will benefit from getting care in a setting that reflects your cultural environment and that is focused on your comfort, your dignity, and your well-being—where you get a sense of being properly cared for.

Having a chronic illness is isolating, and you need to know that you are not alone, that others share your plight, your hopes, and your disappointments. The art of patient navigation in the twenty-first century has added a new dimension to the management of chronic illnesses. Understanding the meaning of a chronic illness is important: it is a disease that is long lasting, usually more than six months, that may or may not go in remission and remain dormant until a flare-up occurs. There are many such illnesses. Diabetes and hypertension are commonly found chronic diseases. Ulcerative colitis, Crohn's disease, some cancers, lupus, and sarcoidosis are other examples. Each is very different and affects different organs and has various modes of management. In most cases of Hepatitis C, the disease does not go into remission but progresses slowly to more severe disease. On average it may take 30 years or more to progress to severe disease. Some people progress toward severe Hepatitis C faster—within 10 years, especially if they have other contributing factors, such as heavy alcohol drinking. Knowledge is power, and educating you and your community on all aspects of Hepatitis C and its management is our mission.

By closely following several patients like Killer Ray who have gone through treatment for Hepatitis C, we have become aware of what "works" and what does not "work" in relation to the disease. In some clinical practices, patients are briefly evaluated, swiftly started on treatment, and just as swiftly taken off treatment. Of course, medicine is an art as well as a science, and there are many situations where it is preferable to discontinue treatment in the best interest of the patient. More often than not, though, treatment is discontinued because of inadequate staffing, insufficient patient information, lack of insurance to continue the treatment, lack of support, or lack of knowledge of how to manage the side effects. Through this book, we hope to guide you, your family, your friends, as well as members of other clinical practices, who perhaps are still apprentices in the very specialized area of chronic Hepatitis C management. While we are attempting to form a health care model to manage Hepatitis C, we also hope to inspire other institutions to follow suit and to optimize the care of patients with chronic illnesses from all cultural and socioeconomic backgrounds.

CHAPTER ONE

A SILENT DISEASE

THE FACTS

- Thirteen years ago Hepatitis C did not even have a name.
- Today, approximately 3.9 million Americans have Hepatitis C.
- Although African Americans only represent 12 percent of the population, 22 percent of people who have Hepatitis C are African Americans.
- Two-thirds of new Hepatitis C cases are due to injection drug use.
- A higher percentage of African-American men than women have the Hepatitis C virus.
- African Americans usually get the Hepatitis C virus called genotype 1, which is the hardest to treat.
- In America, one out of nine African-American men aged 40–49 has Hepatitis C.

Why are so few of us getting diagnosed and treated for Hepatitis C?

- Many of us do not know we are infected.
- Many do not want to know if they are infected.
- Some who know they are infected have been told not to worry about it. There are still some physicians who do not acknowledge the need to evaluate patients and offer them the option of treatment. When will these physicians say in 10 years when their patients suffer from liver failure and need a transplant?
- Treating Hepatitis C is presently not cost-effective because of inadequate health care policies. That is a harsh reality that faces the medical profession and deters physicians from aggressively treating and managing their patients with Hepatitis C. The doctors' reimbursements by HMOs and other health care insurance plans are minimal. In addition, physicians have to pay the high cost of malpractice insurance, as well as the loans many took out to complete medical school. Some doctors just cannot afford the charitable demands this disease puts on the professions. There is dire need for government awareness and intervention, similar to that which is given to HIV centers.

THE IMPORTANCE OF BEING PROACTIVE

In the light of these facts, it is especially important that people with Hepatitis C be proactive. In fact, the very first recommendation made by a National Institute of Health Conference on Hepatitis C, held in 2002, was that the public needed to be educated about the disease. Educating yourself means the following:

- Empowering yourself with knowledge about the disease
- Seeing your primary-care physician, who will perform preliminary tests and refer you to a hepatologist or gastroenterologist, who will treat you immediately, assuming that you have no unforeseen medical complications that would necessitate a delay in treatment
- Lobbying your politicians for prevention programs
- Lobbying for the formation of adequately funded (preferably government-funded) Hepatitis C treatment centers.

By doing these things, you ensure the following:

- You will prevent new infections.
- Doctors will become more proactive and provide treatment when appropriate.
- Your government will fund more educational programs.
- More clinical trials will yield new treatments.
- You will make a difference.

Like Killer Ray, you will share the love. When people with the disease become active on their own behalf, they will conquer Hepatitis C.

HEPATITIS C: THE VIRUS

Hepatitis C is a liver disease caused by a virus that has been named the Hepatitis C virus (HCV). This virus is transmitted from person to person when infected blood comes in contact with noninfected blood. HCV is referred to as the "silent epidemic" because an individual can be infected with the virus for a long time without knowing it. The disease progresses slowly, over years, until a person may have advanced cirrhosis, or scarring, of the liver when he finally finds out he has the virus.

Although Hepatitis C affects all racial and socioeconomic groups, the highest prevalence of the disease is in African-American men between 40 and 60 years old (see Figure 1). African-American males also have a higher rate of hepatocellular carcinoma (see Figure 2). Later in this book we will look at possible reasons for this disparity but, first, three basic questions need to be answered:

- What is the Hepatitis C virus?
- How does the disease act in the infected person?
- What can we do to prevent Hepatitis C, or, if one has already been diagnosed with it, how can we treat it?

Figure 1. Prevalence of Hepatitis C Virus (HCV) infection by age and race/ethnicity—United States, 1988–1994

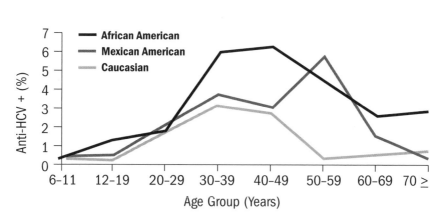

Source: Third National Health and Nutrition Examination Survey, CDC.

Figure 2. Hepatocellular Carcinoma

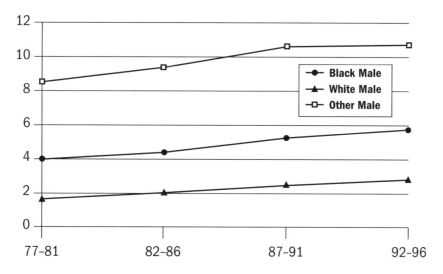

Source: El-Serag and Mason, *NEJM*, 1999

WHAT IS A VIRUS?

Both viruses and bacteria can cause infection, but viruses are different from bacteria. Bacteria are bigger, have their own cells, and behave differently. Most bacterial infections can be treated with antibiotics that kill the bacteria but do not damage the infected cells. A virus is sneakier. It is a very small string of genes that carries a "code" covered by a "protein coat." A virus survives by invading living cells and then using the organisms of the cells to make more virus. You might compare it to Mr. A plugging his TV in his neighbor Mr. B's electrical outlet because Mr. A's house does not have its own working electrical power. Mr. C, who lives on the other side of Mr. B, gets the same idea. Only he comes over and plugs in four air conditioners, two refrigerators, a microwave, and a toaster. Now Mr. B's house, which is supplying all the electricity, has circuit breakers snapping and wires burning up from an overload. Note that Mr. C was causing more damage by using up more electricity. Similarly, some viruses do more damage than others.

When you have the flu, you have a runny nose, cough, and perhaps fever. A virus called influenza type A or B causes these symptoms. Usually, healthy people get better on their own after a few days without any treatment. Other viruses, like HIV, are more serious and attack the entire body's immune system—the system that fights infection.

Vaccines can guard against some viruses. A vaccine is a tiny microscopic amount of a virus injected in a person to protect against infection from the virus. There are, for example, influenza vaccines. All children in the United States are vaccinated against diphtheria, tetanus, Hepatitis A and B. Unfortunately, we do not yet have a vaccine for all viruses. Much work is being done to develop one against HIV. Eventually, we hope and trust, we will also have one to fight against Hepatitis C.

WHAT IS HEPATITIS?

When you see a medical term ending in *itis* (like bronchitis, meningitis, sinusitis, or hepatitis) it usually means an inflammation of a part of the body. Inflammation is a response to injury, usually accompanied by redness and swelling of cells—like a bruise on your skin. Inflammation can be temporary and disappear without permanent damage, or it can be chronic, lasting a long time and possibly causing scar tissue and permanent damage.

Imagine a child falling once or twice on his knees. The knees will have inflammation; they will be red, swollen, painful, possibly bleed a little, form a scab, and, after a while, heal without a scar. Now imagine a different child. This child falls on his knees twice a day, every day for two years. Imagine how much inflammation his poor knees have and imagine what kind of scars he will have from repeated injuries.

Now you understand the main difference between the several forms of hepatitis. The single injury resembles the damage caused by Hepatitis A, and the repeated injuries represent chronic Hepatitis C, a virus that keeps multiplying over many years and eventually destroys many cells and maybe even the entire liver. Hepatitis gets its name from a Greek word that means "liver." Hepatitis means "liver inflammation."

TYPES OF HEPATITIS

There are a number of types of hepatitis. They include the following:

- Viral hepatitis, caused by a virus. This is the most commonly found. The types of viral hepatitis we know now are Hepatitis A, Hepatitis B, Hepatitis C, Hepatitis D, Hepatitis E, and a few more.
- Alcoholic hepatitis, caused by excessive drinking.
- Autoimmune hepatitis, caused by the body's own cells attacking the liver cells.
- Steatohepatitis, also known as "fatty liver," caused by obesity, diabetes or alcohol.
- Drug-induced hepatitis, caused by certain medications.

ACUTE OR CHRONIC HEPATITIS

All forms of viral hepatitis are firstly acute—that is, they last less than six months. All forms can become chronic—that is, they can last more than six months. When a doctor suspects hepatitis, the person being examined should be tested for all of the viruses that cause hepatitis, because those viruses can become contagious (as early as two weeks) and some can cause long-term disease.

A virus that infects liver cells attaches its "spikes" onto the surface of the liver cells, creating a contact point that allows the virus's "bad" gene code to get into the "good" liver cell. Once inside, like the bad neighbor, the virus steals the energy from the normal function of the liver cell and produces more viruses. Over time, this eventually kills the good liver cells, and scar tissue forms on the liver (fibrosis). With the killing of cell after cell, day after day, some viruses can cause severe damage, some in a short period of time, like the Ebola virus, some over a long period of time, like Hepatitis C. Whether the time is short or long, eventually the liver may be so damaged that it stops functioning.

HEPATITIS A

You can get Hepatitis A by eating food or drinking liquid that has come in contact with the human waste of a person infected with Hepatitis A. You may feel very sick for a few days or a few weeks. You may have symptoms such as nausea, vomiting, dark urine, yellow skin, and fatigue, but the body usually gets rid of Hepatitis A on its own, without treatment. To test for Hepatitis A, doctors usually order a blood test for antibodies to the Hepatitis A virus (HAV) and for the liver enzymes levels of alanine aminotransferase (ALT) and bilirubin (the enzyme that causes yellow jaundice). These enzyme levels will most likely be higher than normal. There is no particular treatment for Hepatitis A other than making sure a person drinks plenty of liquids to prevent dehydration.

Risk factors for Hepatitis A listed by the Centers for Disease Control (CDC) are as follows:

- Household contact with people infected with Hepatitis A
- Sexual contact
- Recent international travel in countries where there is a high incidence of Hepatitis A
- Being in contact with infected food handlers working in cafeterias and restaurants.

There is a vaccine available for Hepatitis A. Those who have chronic Hepatitis B or C should be vaccinated for A, because they have a higher risk of getting Hepatitis A or more serious diseases if they get infected.

HEPATITIS B

Hepatitis B virus (HBV) is a more serious virus than the Hepatitis A virus. Hepatitis B is acquired mostly through exchanging blood and body fluids. It is more common than HIV, the virus that causes AIDS. In the United States, 1.2 million people are infected with Hepatitis B. Out of 100 people who are infected, 10 will go on the have chronic infection. With chronic infection comes the risks of developing cirrhosis and liver cancer.

Hepatitis B is a double-stranded deoxyribonucleic acid (DNA) virus. It only occasionally mutates, or changes, its genetic material, so there is a vaccine against Hepatitis B. All children in the United States are offered the Hepatitis B immunization, as are other individuals who are at high risk. Pregnant woman can pass the Hepatitis B virus to their babies. That is why, in the U.S., pregnant women are tested for the virus, and, if positive, their babies at birth are given a shot of Hepatitis B immune globulin (HBIG) to help their immune systems fight the virus if they are infected. According to the CDC, there are 140,000 new cases of Hepatitis B per year.

Risk Factors for Spreading Hepatitis B
There are many risk factors for Hepatitis B. Among them are the following:

- Intravenous drug users sharing needles
- Getting tattoos and body piercing with contaminated needles
- Having unprotected sex with an infected partner
- Vertical transmission (babies born to mothers infected with HBV)
- Cocaine users sharing straws
- Sharing razors, toothbrushes, and nail clippers
- Getting a needle stick or other exposure to blood by health care workers

- Having hemodialysis (patients with end-stage kidney disease on dialysis)
- Traveling internationally to countries where Hepatitis B is common.

Testing for Hepatitis B

Testing for hepatitis starts with the liver enzymes. Some of the tests that may be done are as follows:

- An ALT (alanine aminotransferase) and AST (aspartate aminotransferase) test. ALT and AST are released in the bloodstream when liver cells are destroyed. Therefore, an increase in ALT and AST reflects an inflammation and destruction of those cells.
- A bilirubin test. Bilirubin is a yellow pigment that is usually released from red blood cells and excreted by the liver. When the liver is not working properly, the level rises in the blood.
- A Hepatitis B surface antigen test. If the results of this test are positive, it tells the physician that the patient is infected with the virus.
- A Hepatic B surface antibody test. If this test comes back positive, it shows you have had either prior exposure to the Hepatitis B virus or a previously successful immunization (vaccination) against it.

Various other tests can be ordered to determine the seriousness and stage of the Hepatitis B infection. Tests can determine the following:

- If you are infected
- If you are immune to Hepatitis B
- If you are contagious
- If you are recovering from the infection.

As we stated earlier, only about 10 people out of 100 go on to have chronic infection. Certain cases representing more aggressive forms of the disease may benefit from treatment to stop the progression of liver fibrosis (scarring) to cirrhosis or liver cancer.

Treatment of Hepatitis B consists of using interferon, lamivudine, or adefovir for several months. A person who is infected with chronic Hepatitis B should consult a specialist to determine whether that person might benefit from treatment.

At the very least, those with chronic Hepatitis B should take precautions not to infect others by:

- Practicing safe sex (using condoms)
- Avoiding sharing needles, razors, nail clippers and toothbrushes.

Who Should Be Vaccinated Against Hepatitis B?
These individuals should be vaccinated against Hepatitis B:

- Health care workers
- Police officers
- Firefighters
- Military personnel

- Household members (who live with an infected individual)
- Intravenous drug users
- People with multiple sexual partners
- All persons with HCV and HIV.

HEPATITIS C

The Hepatitis C virus is a single strand RNA (ribonucleic acid) virus of the *Flaviviridiae* family. It is ball-shaped, and is constantly mutating in "quasi species" 5 "genotypes." It

Figure 3. HCV Virus

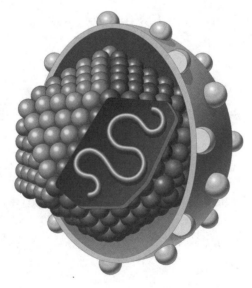

is passed from one person to another by blood-to-blood transmission.

The Centers for Disease Control (CDC) offer the following statistics based on the NHANES survey in the United States:

- About 4 million Americans are infected with Hepatitis C.
- Hepatitis C is the number one reason for liver transplantations.
- Hepatitis C infects 1.8 percent of the U.S. population.
- Hepatitis C infects 11 percent of African-American males aged 40–49.
- 85 percent of those infected with Hepatitis C develop chronic infection (compared to 10 percent with Hepatitis B).
- 20 percent of those infected develop cirrhosis, among which 4–8 percent develop liver cancer.

The estimate that 4 million Americans are infected with Hepatitis C is probably a gross underestimate, because it was based on a survey of household populations. It did not include prison inmates, homeless persons, institutionalized persons, or veterans. In these subpopulations, the NIH (National Institutes of Health), in June 2002, established that the rates of infection ranged from 15 to 90 percent. The highest prevalence (70–90 percent) was found in intravenous drug users and hemophiliacs who were treated with contaminated blood products prior to 1992.

The Hepatitis C virus was not discovered until 1989, when Dr. Michael Houghton identified it. In the early 1980s, the virus had not been identified and was known only as "non-A non-B virus." In 1990, shortly after Dr. Houghton's discovery, a test was developed to detect exposure to Hepatitis C virus.

While we now know the genetic makeup or "genome" of the virus, we have not yet been able to develop a vaccine. The main reason is the elusiveness of the virus— it constantly mutates (changes its genetic material) into quasi-species. To understand quasi-species, imagine the following: You are a detective looking for a skinny, tall man wearing a yellow hat. But every time you come close to catching him, he is wearing a different colored hat. You know the man's features and general description, but he changes hats to mislead you.

The Hepatitis C virus is like the hat-changing man. The virus comes in different genotypes: 1a, 1b, 2a, 2b, 3, 4, 5, 6. Each genotype has a different arrangement of genes. Like cousins in a family, one is a fast runner, one is a good jumper, one is a good pianist, and one is a good dancer. These cousins are all in the same family but behave differently. So it is with Hepatitis C. We know that certain genotypes of Hepatitis C are more difficult to treat. We also know that in different parts of the world there are different concentrations of genotypes. In Europe, there are more people infected with genotype 2 and 3, which is the easiest to treat. In the United States, 72 percent of those infected with Hepatitis C have genotype 1a and 1b, the most difficult to treat. Also, certain genotypes progress to a more advanced disease in a shorter amount of time.

Risk Factors for Hepatitis C
There are as many risk factors linked to Hepatitis C as there are the Hepatitis B. Among them are the following:

- Intravenous illicit drug use with shared needles (including history of one-time use)
- Getting tattoos and body piercing with contaminated needles
- Cocaine use with shared straws (even only once)
- Sharing razors, toothbrushes, and nail clippers
- Having a needle stick or other exposure to blood by health care workers
- Having had hemodialysis (i.e., patients on dialysis with end-state kidney disease)
- Having had a blood transfusion or organ transplant prior to 1990
- Being one of the 5 percent of children born to infected mothers
- Participating in high-risk sexual behavior
- Being a Vietnam War veteran
- Being an HIV-positive individual
- Serving time in jail
- Being from countries where routine vaccination was done with shared syringes.

Who should get tested for Hepatitis C?

- All those with prior risk factors
- All sexual partners of infected people (at least once)
- All patients with abnormal liver enzymes
- All patients with a history of alcohol abuse because of its frequent association with illicit drug use.

What Are the Symptoms of Chronic Hepatitis C?

Most people with Hepatitis C feel fine until they develop the advanced disease—that is, until their liver develops cirrhosis or significant scar tissue.

Symptoms of Hepatitis C include the following:

- Fatigue
- Depression and anxiety. Some studies report as many as 25–30 percent of patients with Hepatitis C are depressed compared to 9.5 percent in the general population.
- Joint and muscle pains. Several patients who thought they had some form of arthritis were found to have Hepatitis C.
- Nausea and loss of appetite.

If you have any of these complaints you need to be evaluated by your primary-care physician or at your local Emergency Room.

Hepatitis C and African Americans
As shown in Figure 1, the number of people diagnosed with HCV is relatively higher among African Americans than among Caucasians or Hispanics. In the light of that fact, the National Medical Association (NMA), representing 25,000 African-American and Caribbean physicians, has issued a statement acknowledging the urgent need to promote prevention of viral hepatitis in the African-American community by

- Providing health education in school about liver wellness
- Getting more African-American subjects and researchers recruited for clinical trials
- Starting advocacy groups modeled on those that rally for HIV/AIDS to focus on issues related to hepatitis.

Dr. Alpha Banks, an African-American hepatologist from Greenbelt, Maryland, has tried to examine the cause of the racial disparities related to hepatitis. She suspects that, at the time of diagnosis, her African-American patients are more likely to have been infected longer than her Caucasian patients. One possible reason is that African Americans are less likely to be insured and therefore have less access to treatment. They are also less likely to have received Hepatitis A and B vaccines. People who do not have much money or education are more likely to participate in risky behaviors, such as home tattooing, intravenous drug use, and unprotected sex. The National Institutes of Health (NIH) has addressed these issues by funding several research proposals looking at progression and treatment of Hepatitis C.

African Americans account for 12 percent of the U.S. population and 14 percent of intravenous drug users; therefore, they do not inject illicit drugs more often than the rest of the population. But they may do it less safely by sharing contaminated needles or other paraphernalia of illicit drug use. Efforts to stop illegal drug use are very noble, but we must also face the reality that there are people who will continue using heroin or cocaine and should be protected from infection. The Harm Reduction Coalition (*www.harmreduction.org*) has addressed this issue and has published several pamphlets on the safety practices of drug users. The coalition should be commended for directing efforts at preventing the transmission of this virus.

Recent surveys suggest that there are distinct racial and ethnic differences with respect to the prevalence, response to therapy, and complications of chronic Hepatitis C infection of African Americans compared with Caucasians.

African Americans represent about 12 or 13 percent of the population in the United States. Yet the group accounts for 22 percent of U.S. citizens chronically infected with Hepatitis C. Once infected, African Americans, among whom genotype 1—the hardest form of the disease to treat—is the most common, appear to be more susceptible to chronic infection. African Americans were also found to have less ability to suppress Hepatitis C with antiviral therapy. On the positive side, despite the higher chance of developing chronic infection, African Americans seem to exhibit slower rates of progression to cirrhosis and advanced liver disease.

Researchers of HCV find a higher percentage of African Americans infected than Caucasians (and more African-American men than African-American women). Research also shows that infected African-American men and women do not respond as well to treatment or transplant as Caucasian men and women do, and have higher mortality rates, as shown in Figure 4.

Much research remains to be done to understand why African Americans do not respond as well to treatment. We know from our experience that compliance to treatment is not an issue. Our population is brave and determined to fight the disease. We take the time to follow up adequately through treatment, personal calls, and frequent visits. Researchers are now looking at insulin resistance as a mechanism that might be influenced by interferon treatment. Other researchers are looking at different levels of certain chemicals, called cytokines, which occur naturally in the body and help to protect it.

Obviously we need more clinical trials to find answers and develop treatment options that best serve the needs of our African-American population. We need to establish different criteria for evaluating drops in white blood cells

Figure 4. HCV Mortality Rate per 100,000 Population, 1982–1995

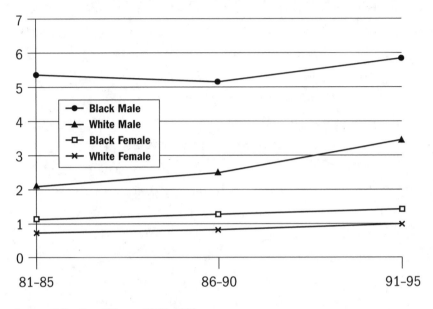

Source: El-Serag and Mason, *NEJM*, 1999

when we know that our African-American patients already have lower numbers of white blood cells to begin with. Some of the research has just begun and more is needed.

The most recent data tells us that patients who have blood transfusions no longer have to be concerned about being infected with HCV. At the same time, the number of people getting the Hepatitis C virus through sexual transmission rose by 3 percent, and intravenous drug users rose to 68 percent of the HCV population.

Lack of public knowledge about Hepatitis C only makes the risk of infection greater. Already, just over 4 million Americans are infected with the Hepatitis C virus

(HCV). That's almost the entire population of Chicago. Conservative data indicates that the number of Hepatitis C cases amounts to about 1.8 percent of the U.S. population. Three out of four people with the illness do not even know that they have it.

There are five times more Hepatitis C cases in the U.S. than cases of Parkinson's disease. And Americans are, astoundingly, 10 times more likely to be diagnosed with Hepatitis C than with multiple sclerosis. And yet, there are no telethons, no marathons, and little public outcry for more information and research on Hepatitis C.

Hepatitis C sufferers are not just found in the United States. It is a global problem. The World Health Organization (WHO) estimates that Hepatitis C infects 3 percent of the world population—a far higher rate than the 1.8 percent of Americans coping with the problem. An estimated 400 million people around the world are infected with HCV, compared to 20 million with HIV/AIDS.

HEPATITIS EPIDEMIC AMONG VETERANS

Some researchers attribute the alarmingly high incidence of HCV infection among veterans and ex-prisoners to the disproportionate number of African-Americans in poverty, incarcerated, and in the military. A 1997 study of patients at Veterans Administration (VA) hospitals revealed a disturbing trend. In 1991, there were 6,612 cases of HCV at the locations surveyed. The next year, the count rose to 8,365—21 percent more. And at the conclusion of the four-year study, HCV patients had increased 286 percent from the original number, to 18,854.

While this study of veterans at VA institutions was revealing, a more shocking concept is what the actual figures may be when you take into account the huge number of veterans who never check in to such VA facilities and the hundreds of thousands of war veterans who are homeless.

Given the high rates of HCV among African Americans and veterans, the need for continued testing of those at highest risk is crucial. If you are in a high-risk group, you should insist on getting tested for HCV. If you have been associated with any of the risk factors mentioned, you should also be tested. If you have a primary-care physician, get tested there. If you do not, HCV tests are available in hospital emergency rooms.

If you are in a high-risk group, you should insist on getting tested for HCV. If you have been associated with any of the factors mentioned, you should also be tested.

FINDING CARE

If you show symptoms, or have one or several of the risk factors listed above, it is urgently important that you visit your primary-care physician, who will perform the

Many scientists believe the high infection rate among veterans is a result of the exposure to so many Hepatitis C risk factors while in the military. These include:

- Exposure to tainted blood during combat and combat training
- Medical care under unsanitary conditions
- Short supply of medical equipment for vaccines
- Transfusions before blood was screened in 1992
- Service duty in areas of high rates of infection, including Asia and North Africa
- High rate of drug use
- Crowded living conditions
- Tattoos.

preliminary test. If that test is positive, your primary-care physician will refer you to a specialist, who will treat you with interferon and ribavirin, currently the treatment of choice for Hepatitis C.

A private office is often a good place to be treated. Usually you trust your doctor and have a good, friendly relationship with his or her staff. That is important because you, the doctor, and his staff are all members of the same team, whose single goal is your best health. If you do not have a primary-care doctor, you can get tested in an emergency room.

Another very good place to be treated is a "center of excellence," a hospital that best serves the community by offering treatment at the cutting edge of knowledge, and with staff specifically trained to address all aspects of disease management. This is important since you want your clinicians to be knowledgeable, compassionate, and attuned to your needs, which may be similar to, but are always slightly different from, those of other patients.

The additional advantage of being treated in a center of excellence that is well staffed is that your health care provider is available, and that he or she will call you back and will follow up. You should feel as if *you* are important and that all your tests will be reviewed with the utmost attention and concern for your safety and health.

CHAPTER TWO

THE IMPORTANCE OF A HEALTHY LIVER

What we call normal daily body functions depend on the cooperation between the body's various organs and systems of operation. Certain functions, such as breathing and digesting food, require the cooperation of many organs. Other functions are performed by one specific organ. Some organs, and even the various cells of the body, perform many functions.

The liver may be the most fascinating of the body's organs—it performs over fifty different distinct functions.

WHAT THE LIVER IS AND DOES

The liver is the largest organ in the body, ordinarily weighing about 3.5 pounds. It measures about 8 to 9 inches in length and 4 to 5 inches in width. It is located in the abdominal area of the body, just beneath the diaphragm of the stomach.

Figure 5. Anatomy of the liver, gall bladder and stomach

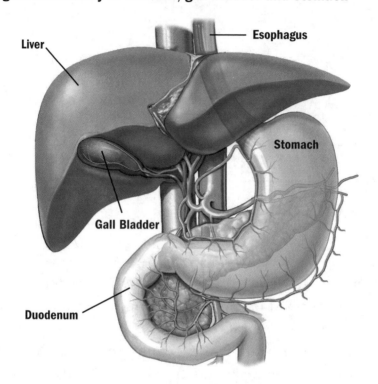

While most of us know where the liver is, few of us understand what it does. The location part is easy—the liver is in the abdomen, tucked below the ribs on the right side. But *what* it does is more complicated.

Let us start at the tiniest micro level. The liver is a mass of a few *billion* tiny cells that manufacture chemicals needed by the body and destroy chemicals that are unneeded or harmful to the body.

While those housekeeping tasks are going on, the liver works also as a *productive* organ, converting nutrients absorbed from the bowel into sophisticated new chemicals. As an example, the liver can turn digested foods like cornflakes into substances that make our blood clot when we cut ourselves.

The multitasking liver performs still another essential job: the liver cells break down and eliminate waste products of body metabolism and toxic chemicals absorbed from the bowel. Because the liver's functions *are* complex, it is possible for one function of the liver to be interfered with while others proceed normally.

Blood comes to the liver from the stomach, spleen, pancreas, and intestines. The liver helps to regulate the blood volume of the body by storing blood and releasing it through the hepatic vein. The liver can hold up to a pint of blood at a time, an amount equal to about 13 percent of the body's total blood supply.

The anatomy of the system is reasonably simple After blood vessels have gathered their nutrients from the bowel, they channel the blood directly to the liver through the large "portal vein." The liver then filters important nutrients and gets rid of unwanted blood toxins, sending them into the bowel through the bile duct.

Much of what goes into the bile duct is waste intended for discharge from the body, but the file itself contains chemicals that help with digestion. In the gall bladder, a small organ attached to the bile duct, bile is stored and then released back into the duct on cues from the stomach.

The liver forms and secretes about 800 to 1200 ml of bile daily. Bile is formed from bile salts and .water, bile pigments, lecithin, and cholesterol. Bile salts are important in the intestinal phase of digestion because the salts work as detergents to emulsify fats. Cholesterol is made soluble by bile salts and lecithin. Interestingly, the body recycles about 80 percent of the bile salts in the small intestines, and then returns them to the liver.

The liver serves a key role in the metabolism of carbohydrates, fats, and proteins. For instance, it stores glycogen, which maintains blood sugar consistency. The liver is also center stage in the metabolism of fats; it oxidizes fatty acids, it synthesizes fats from glucose, and it forms lipoproteins, which combine proteins with fatty-like substances.

Another function of the liver is to store and allow absorption of fat-soluble vitamins such as A, E, and K. Vitamins are not produced in the body; they must come from nutrition, pills, or injections. Each vitamin plays an important role. Vitamin K, for example, helps form globulin, which is needed for the coagulation of blood.

The liver is a key organ in your body's self-defense system. It changes or detoxifies many harmful substances into forms that your body can safely eliminate. It controls the concentrations of various substances and also detoxifies certain end-products of digestion. Further, the liver plays an important role in regulating estrogen levels by excreting excess estrogen through the bile. Finally, the liver helps provide heat for the body.

A gradual decline in liver function is part of the normal aging process. As long as there is no disease, this declining function does not present a problem because the liver has a tremendous amount of built-in reserve.

WHAT HAPPENS WHEN THE LIVER IS DAMAGED?

With functions so diverse and complex, it is remarkable that the liver serves us so well. Failure of this organ is less common than failure of the other vital organs, but disease can strike and produce symptoms.

The early symptoms of some liver diseases are nausea, lack of appetite, and jaundice, or yellowing, of the skin. The symptoms are most likely to occur in cases of Hepatitis A and B than in C, but they may appear in advanced cases of Hepatitis C.

The jaundice is caused by the back up of bile. More severe symptoms, such as bleeding, fluid retention, and coma, are seen when other organ systems fail from lack of needed chemicals and from accumulation of toxins.

Hepatitis, cirrhosis, and cancer are the most common diseases affecting the liver. Hepatitis is an inflammation of liver cells caused by such agents as viruses, drugs, alcohol, and poisons. Hepatitis can be very mild and free of symptoms or can be severe and lead to liver failure.

Cirrhosis is an advanced stage of scarring caused by chronic liver inflammation. In cirrhosis, dead liver cells are replaced by scar tissue. If enough liver cells die, the result is liver failure and often death. Nevertheless, some people live with cirrhosis for ten years or even more.

The most common causes of cirrhosis are alcohol

Figure 6. Healthy liver and cirrhotic liver

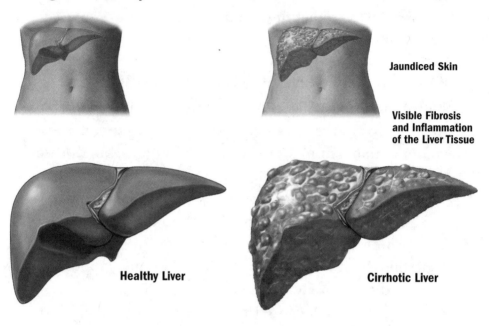

Jaundiced Skin

Visible Fibrosis
and Inflammation
of the Liver Tissue

Healthy Liver

Cirrhotic Liver

abuse and infection with the Hepatitis C virus. Cancer frequently involves the liver, but it usually spreads to the organ from other sites. Cancer that *starts* in the liver is most commonly seen in patients who have chronic viral hepatitis.

If the liver is not properly performing its functions, the rest of the body will soon be affected by the lack of nutrients and by the excess waste products present in the blood. (An unhealthy liver does not detoxify substances as rapidly or as completely as a healthy liver. Slower detoxification results in more toxic substances circulating in the body.)

Unchanged or partially changed toxins are not easily eliminated and instead pass from the liver into the body. Eventually, the toxins are stored in fatty body tissue, including the brain and central nervous system cells. Stored toxins may be slowly released into the blood, contributing to many chronic illnesses.

In today's world of processed foods and pollution, toxic substances exist almost everywhere. They are in the food you eat, the water you drink (chemicals from fertilizers and pesticides, and other additives such as colorings and preservatives), and the air you breathe (from automobile emissions, pesticides, and industrial pollutants). A healthy liver is able to rid you of these toxins along with those your body produces. An unhealthy liver cannot.

ALCOHOL AND RECREATIONAL DRUGS

Repeated exposure to chemicals and toxins in food, water, and elsewhere from the environment increases the burden on your liver. Alcohol and recreational drugs directly weaken the liver's ability to function, by overloading the liver's capacity to detoxify them.

The liver processes everything a person consumes, including alcohol. When a person has a drink, the alcohol is absorbed directly through the wall of the stomach and intestine into the bloodstream, where it is distributed rapidly throughout the body. The alcohol changes the function of each cell it enters.

Because many of us consider ourselves to be nondrinkers or social drinkers, I am going to assume that you are not currently an alcoholic. But even social drinkers may not consciously notice just how much we actually drink at that occasional wedding reception, birthday party, or office celebration. Nor do most of us consciously consider that the margarita in our hand is going to affect the organs in our body.

Just keep in mind that your liver is the only organ that processes alcohol and that only a limited quantity of alcohol can be detoxified within a given period of time. In the meantime, the excess alcohol affects your brain, heart, muscles, and other tissues in the body.

When the liver has too much alcohol to handle, normal liver function may be interrupted, leading to a chemical imbalance. If the liver is required, hour after hour, to detoxify alcohol, liver cells may be destroyed or altered, resulting in fat deposits (fatty liver) and, more seriously, either inflammation (alcoholic hepatitis), and/or permanent scarring (cirrhosis).

FATTY LIVER

Fatty liver is the excessive accumulation of fat inside the liver cells. Fatty liver is the most common liver disorder caused by alcohol. It results in your liver enlarging, eventually causing you to feel upper abdominal discomfort on the right side.

ALCOHOLIC HEPATITIS

Alcoholic hepatitis is an acute inflammation of the liver, accompanied by the destruction of individual liver cells and scarring. Symptoms may include fever, jaundice, an increased white blood cell count, an enlarged, tender liver, and spiderlike veins in the skin.

ALCOHOLIC CIRRHOSIS

Alcoholic cirrhosis is the destruction of normal liver tissue, leaving nonfunctioning scar tissue. Symptoms may include those of alcoholic hepatitis in addition to the following:

- Hypertension in the portal vein of the liver
- Enlarged spleen
- Accumulation of fluid
- Kidney failure
- Confusion
- Liver cancer.

Symptoms of alcohol-induced liver disease depend on how much and how long a person has been drinking alcohol. The following are the most common symptoms of alcohol-induced liver disease, though symptoms will appear in different combinations from one patient to another. Symptoms may include the following:

- Fatigue
- Confusion

- Loss of appetite
- Lowered resistance to infections
- Enlarged liver
- Fever
- Jaundice—yellowing of the skin and eyes
- Increased white blood cell count
- Spiderlike veins in the skin
- Portal hypertension
- Enlarged spleen
- Fluid buildup and swelling of the abdomen
- Intestinal bleeding
- Brain dysfunction
- Kidney failure.

More than three-quarters of your liver cells may be nonfunctioning before you notice any symptoms, and by then it may be too late to do anything about it. The symptoms of alcohol-induced liver disease may also resemble other medical conditions or problems. So it is important to have regular checkups with a doctor, who will be able to detect early signs of liver disease through physical examinations and blood tests.

ALCOHOL AND LIVER DAMAGE

Let us begin with how you can prevent liver damage, and perhaps prevent Hepatitis C as well. To prevent liver damage, you have to keep your eyes on how much you drink. Your proper alcohol limit depends on your body weight, gender, and other factors. For example, women are more susceptible than men to alcohol-related liver damage. If your total weekly consumption of alcohol exceeds 14 "drinks" (an average of more than two drinks per day) serious damage may be done to the liver, regardless of whether you are female or male.

No one alcoholic beverage is safer or better than any other. It is the amount of alcohol present in a drink that matters, not the type of drink. We are define "one drink" in terms of the equivalents listed below:

- One can/12 ounces (341 ml) beer
- One glass/5 ounces (142 ml) wine
- Less than 2 shots of any "real" liquor—that is, about 1 ½ ounces (43 ml) spirits.

Each of the above has the same effect on the liver whether taken alone or diluted. Mixing soda with the wine to make a spritzer or letting the ice melt in that whiskey sour will not weaken the alcohol's effect.

If caught early, minor liver damage can be reversed if a person stops drinking alcohol. When there is no alcohol in the bloodstream, slow but marked improvement in the liver cells will allow the liver to return to normal. The liver has tremendous capacity to regenerate itself. If necessary, a doctor may also suggest that a person whose liver is impaired be treated with new drug therapies. In many cases, these treatments allow people to live normal lives.

Alcohol-related diseases vary in severity. Fatty liver and

mild alcoholic hepatitis can be cured; however, advanced alcoholic hepatitis can result in serious illness.

When cirrhosis develops, the structure of the liver is permanently damaged. The symptoms, signs, and outcome of cirrhosis depend on its severity and whether or not it is accompanied by severe fatty liver and/or alcoholic hepatitis.

The combination of these forms of alcohol-related liver disease may cause illness and, sometimes, death. Look after your liver and, if you choose to drink alcohol, have no more than two drinks a day.

Mixing alcohol and medications also damages the liver.

ALCOHOL AND HEPATITIS C

If you have Hepatitis C or any other liver disease, it is best that you do not drink at all. Discuss with your doctor whether it is possible for you to have an occasional drink. Only your doctor, who knows your exact condition, can give you specific advice.

Also, check with your doctor about whether the medications you take for Hepatitis C mean that you should drink no alcohol at all. That includes over-the-counter drugs as well. It may be dangerous for you to take alcohol with many everyday drugs, such as acetaminophen, commonly found in nonaspirin pain relievers (such as Tylenol, Motrin, and Advil). In short, consult your doctor before you drink alcohol with any medication.

HEPATITIS C AND DRUGS

So what if you do not consume much alcohol but are doing drugs? Almost any medication, including some herbal preparations and illicit drugs, make it harder for the liver to function normally. Some common prescription medications known to have such negative effects are listed below:

- Nonsteroidal anti-inflammatory drugs
- Antibiotics
- Cholesterol-lowering statins
- Antituberculosis drugs.

Many herbs or homeopathic treatments, including ephedra, chaparral, Alchemilla, Scutellaria, and shark cartilage, have been reported to cause elevations in liver enzyme levels. Use of anabolic steroids, amphetamines, cocaine, crack, ecstasy, PCP, glue, or solvents may also injure the liver.

The liver performs functions for your body that are basic to your good health; functions such as getting rid of toxins. If the liver cannot perform its key functions, the accumulating toxins will cause disease. In the next chapter, we will talk about what to expect after your doctor tells you that you have, or may have, Hepatitis C.

CHAPTER THREE

FACING THE DIAGNOSIS: "WHY DIDN'T ANYONE EVER TELL ME?"

People who have just learned that they have a serious illness usually react with shock. Let us take a look at the common scenario. You were just told that you have a serious illness when you thought you were in relatively good health. During the days that follow, you will experience fear and anxiety. After all, your whole life has hit a sudden barrier.

Once the shock wears off you will ask a big question: why me? If the disease is caused by an infection like Hepatitis C, you will wonder how and when you became infected.

Other questions will flash through your head: What did I do wrong? Who did this to me? Was it my own fault? Why didn't my doctor tell me years ago?

Shock will shift to anger at yourself and at those who might have communicated the disease to you. There is no end of anger—anger at the world, at the blood transfusion, at the sexual partner who infected you, at yourself for trying heroin, at your friend for sharing a contaminated cocaine straw, even at God for letting it happen.

Then there might be denial: "I feel fine. There must be a mistake. I want a second opinion."

At this stage, too, fear of the unknown future will set in—fear of the complications of the disease, fear of being discovered by friends and stigmatized (blamed for reckless activity), fear of being rejected by your boyfriend or girlfriend.

Some people will experience depression. The signs of depression are feeling worthless and hopeless, losing interest in pleasurable activities such as sex, eating, or playing ball. There may also be physical signs such as tiredness, headaches, and other symptoms.

Here are some of the worries we have heard expressed by our own patients:

- What will my future be like?
- What will happen to me?
- Could I die from this?
- How long will I live?

People seem to have to go through all those painful stages—shock, anger, denial, acceptance, and finally courage—before they can allow acceptance to set in. Acceptance has its own batch of questions: the crucial one is "Okay, I have Hepatitis C. What do I do now?"

WHY PEOPLE GET DIAGNOSED LATE

One obstacle to acceptance of the Hepatitis C diagnosis is that people blame themselves for not getting diagnosed earlier. But there are many good reasons why you may not have known that you were infected until now:

· If you had one of the risk factors, such as a blood transfusion, in 1975, or once snorted cocaine at a party back in 1976, you may not have told your doctor. You may even have forgotten or wanted to forget.

· If you were infected before 1990, the Hepatitis C virus wasn't yet discovered.

· You may be one of the many people whose routine blood tests are negative but who are nevertheless carrying the disease.

· You may not have gotten a specific Hepatitis C antibody test. (Doctors only test persons who have risk factors.)

· If you weren't screened for Hepatitis C, even though you had risk factors, you won't know if you have the disease.

· You may be one of the many who don't feel sick until the disease is fairy advanced.

You can see that there are lots of reasons why the diagnosis of Hepatitis C can come as a great shock.

Particularly important here is that, because the symptoms of even the acute phase of the disease are often mild, in many people they go unnoticed. Few people with acute-phase Hepatitis C experience yellow jaundice or recall ever having any symptoms of liver disease. The disease progresses slowly over many years. Some people do not find out they have Hepatitis C until their liver is already failing. By that time, chances for successful treatment are much lower than they would have been had the disease been found at an earlier stage.

Absence of symptoms is not the only problem. People sometimes fail to get diagnosed because of selective memory or because they are reluctant to share aspects of their behaviors or lifestyle that they think may cause them to be stigmatized. Misunderstanding by African Americans of the potential dangers of Hepatitis C causes many people with risk factors to go without testing and treatment, according to a landmark survey commissioned by the American Gastroenterological Association (AGA).

To dispel the myths about Hepatitis C, we need to face the facts. Even though far more Americans are infected by hepatitis and will probably die from it in the next decade than from HIV/AIDS, the AGA survey reveals that 8 out of 10 Americans believe AIDS is a serious threat while only half of them consider the Hepatitis C virus to be on par with HIV. The survey is part of AGA's "Be Hepatitis C SMART" (Shattering Myths and Reinforcing Truths) campaign to educate the public and health care providers about the prevention, diagnosis, and treatment of Hepatitis C.

Here are some of the myths and kinds of misinformation that the AGA survey revealed, in average Americans *and* in medical professionals:

- 32 percent of Americans mistakenly believe the Hepatitis C virus can be spread through fecal contamination, water, or food.
- 42 percent do not know that Hepatitis C can be contracted through *any* contact with infected blood.
- 12 percent of those surveyed believe that people like themselves do not get HCV.
- 34 percent of Americans are not aware that there are prescription drugs that can treat Hepatitis C, which means the majority of people with the disease do not get the help they need.

HEPATITIS C AND ILLEGAL INTRAVENOUS DRUGS

The greatest number of cases of Hepatitis C are caused by the use of illegal intravenous (IV) drugs. Seven out of 10 users of IV drugs have Hepatitis C. You are considered a user if you used IV drugs yesterday or 10 years ago. If you used IV drugs at all, you are still at risk for Hepatitis C. To make matters worse, because there are seldom symptoms for HCV, as many as 85 percent of those who have the disease are unaware that they have it. Otherwise healthy individuals, who have gone on to successful careers and to raise families, are unable to accept the notion that something they did 20 or more years ago is coming back to haunt them.

If you have ever used illegal IV drugs, here are the facts: The average person with chronic Hepatitis C has a blood concentration of the virus amounting to 2 million particles per milliliter of whole blood. That means 2,000 particles of virus in as much blood as can be found on the head of a stickpin.

Given that significant concentration, people who think they can sanitize or sterilize needles by wiping or rinsing them clean are sadly mistaken. What drug users fail to recognize is that such efforts to clean needles do not work because the internal chamber of the syringe does not get irrigated or washed and the exterior parts of the syringe are not cleansed in the process. Cleaning a needle requires a concentrated solution, such as hydrogen peroxide, to inactivate the virus enough to reduce the risk of its transmission. And even that is not nearly as effective as true sterilization.

That is why you are at risk if you have ever used IV drugs. It is also why you especially need to seek out treatment.

FIRST STEPS TOWARD BEING TREATED

When you have been diagnosed with the Hepatitis C virus, you need to know where you go next. The first step is to rely on your health care professional. If the first doctor you talk to does not seem genuinely interested in you, is not knowledgeable about your disease, and cannot explain it to you in terms that are clear to you, do not be shy about getting a second opinion. This is your life we are talking about. Some new patients enroll in Moving

Forward, a support group for those chronically infected with HCV.

This is a good time to get to know your doctor and make sure you get the right care for your condition. You might want to ask a few questions, such as:

- What is the level of Hepatitis C virus in your blood?
- What do all of the test results mean?
- What are the results and implications of the genotype test?
- How much experience has your doctor had in dealing with patients infected with HCV?

EVEN THE STARS . . .

While some lifestyles definitely raise the risk of Hepatitis C, it is important to know that this disease crosses gender and racial lines. For those involved in risky behaviors, the threat is real. It does not matter if you are a poor, unemployed homeless man or woman, or an affluent individual with a spacious condominium overlooking the shores of southern France. It can happen to anyone.

Naomi Judd, a popular country singer, has been very active in raising awareness of Hepatitis C. The effects of the disease—headaches, flulike symptoms, and fatigue—forced her to retire from the popular country music duo, The Judds, in 1991. That left daughter Wynonna to go it alone.

After taking an antiviral drug for approximately a year, Ms. Judd's condition stabilized. An accomplished performer for many years, she is also a former registered nurse. She had never done IV drugs, she had always been monogamous, and she had never been drunk—so it is possible she contracted the disease through an accidental needle stick. In rare instances, these types of incidents continue to occur and are still being reported.

Hospitals and clinics have really stepped up safety precautions for their workers in the wake of HIV/AIDS transmission, but many accidental transmissions of HIV and HCV remain undetected.

ORDINARY PEOPLE

No single pattern defines people who have been diagnosed with HCV. Here are some stories created to represent typical patients diagnosed with Hepatitis C:

"Jerome" Drank

Jerome was a 43-year-old homeless man who managed to live on the street, going from soup kitchen to shelters, and drinking whatever he could, whenever he could, until one day he found himself vomiting blood on the street in a back alley of Harlem. He was scared. He claimed he was never sick one day in his life, that he was strong like an ox and must have eaten bad food. He was brought into the emergency room, evaluated, and admitted to the intensive care unit, where endoscopy was performed and he was found to have bleeding esophageal varices (enlarged veins in the tube leading from the mouth to the stomach). Those veins were banded. The bleeding stopped. Jerome received blood transfusions.

In addition to being an alcoholic, he was found to have Hepatitis C, a double "hit" to his liver. His liver had advanced cirrhosis. This was a serious warning. His doctors told him how important it was for him to follow up this visit with further evaluation and to stop drinking because the next time he might not be so lucky; he might not make it to the hospital or the bleeding might not stop.

Jerome was directed to join a rehab program. But he chose to continue drinking despite the doctors' warnings. Three months later, he was carried in again, vomiting blood profusely this time, his belly swollen up like a balloon (ascites). He became jaundiced and confused. Doctors were able to stop the bleeding, but Jerome went into a coma and died. He was a victim of Hepatitis C and alcohol abuse. He had never known he had Hepatitis C until his first hospital admission.

"Denise" Has Sickle Cell Anemia

Denise is 32-year-old African-American lady who works as a legal secretary. She has a disease called sickle cell anemia, like many other African Americans. Her condition has been stable for years. Her doctors have been keeping Denise on medication that prevents her from having a sickle cell crisis. She has not needed a transfusion since she was 15 years old. She has been taking care of herself. But recently her doctor told her that her liver chemistry was a little abnormal. Denise was referred to a liver clinic, and, during her evaluation, it was discovered that she had Hepatitis C. Denise may have had the disease since she was only one year old, when she received her first blood transfusion. After taking a liver biopsy from her, we found out that Denise's liver has stage 3 fibrosis. That is fairly advanced disease.

Denise is a challenging case: the new combination therapy that we offer to other patients is not safe for her because of her anemia. At age 32, her liver is already at stage 3 of damage. She may have cirrhosis at age 42 and may or may not develop complications. Denise knows that we are looking out for her. We assure her that we are consulting experts in the field, all over the country where research is going on—experts who specialize in difficult cases. We also reassure her that we are keeping her in mind for future therapies, hoping that a treatment is found soon enough to either arrest the damage or, hopefully, reverse it.

For years Denise thought her biggest challenge was sickle cell anemia. All of a sudden Hepatitis C may one day threaten her life. She is sticking with us, she trusts that we are monitoring her safety, and she reads and searches the Internet herself. We like that patients keep informed. The more you know and understand, the better you can help your doctor to guide you, and the better you can help yourself.

"Patricia Had a C-Section"

"I have been to doctors regularly for the last 25 years and nobody ever told me I had liver disease. It must be a mistake. I want a second opinion. . . ." So said Patricia, a 52-year-old African-American lady who had a Caesarian section (C-section) in 1972. Because the operation can be painful, Patricia was anesthetized ("put to sleep") before it began. She does not recall being given a blood transfusion, but she remembers being anemic after the operation.

Patricia did not know she had liver disease. She only drinks alcohol on Christmas and New Year's Eve, never did any illicit drug, and has no tattoos. She most likely had a blood transfusion at the time of her C-section. Her liver enzymes are normal. She found out she had Hepatitis C when she went to donate blood during a blood drive at her church. She then had a liver biopsy, which showed stage 3 of fibrosis. She is genotype 2, which means she will only need six months of treatment. She has been in treatment for 10 weeks and has been tolerating it well.

"Jimmy" Partied at a Fraternity Gathering in 1969

Jimmy is a 57-year-old African-American lawyer, married with children, and in good health. For the last 25 years he has maintained a healthy lifestyle by exercising almost daily and by playing tennis. His biggest concern had been trying to avoid developing diabetes, which his mother, aunt and uncle, and grandmother all had. As an educated man, Jimmy had read that obesity and family history would predispose him to developing diabetes, and he was determined to do all he could to avoid getting it. At age 32, being overweight (he weighed 245 pounds while measuring 5 feet 10 inches tall), he visited his family doctor. He asked the doctor to direct him in losing weight and to test for possible signs of diabetes. Jimmy's fasting blood sugar level was normal. Since that visit to the doctor, Jimmy lost 38 pounds and maintained a trim body.

In 2001, Jimmy changed law firms, and his insurance coverage was different. He had to get himself a new primary-care physician, so he scheduled an appointment with one. His new physician checked his medical history by asking him numerous questions about the following risk factors:

- Risk for cardiovascular disease, diabetes, colon cancer, and prostate cancer
- Cigarette smoking
- Past or current use of illicit drugs
- Unsafe sex with multiple partners
- Sex with a steady partner who has Hepatitis C
- Tattoos and/or body piercings
- Personal items, such as razors or toothbrushes, shared with others
- Mother with Hepatitis C at the time of one's birth
- Blood transfusion before blood screening took effect in July 1992
- Treatment for blood clot problems with a product made before 1987

- Dialysis or an organ transplant
- Work in a health care environment where there was a risk of needle sticks and sharp pricks.

Jimmy's doctor explained that, based on Jimmy's history of cocaine use in 1969, he would want to rule out any exposure to Hepatitis B or C. The doctor ordered the appropriate test. Lo and behold, Jimmy's blood tested positive for the antibody to Hepatitis C, which meant that he had been exposed to the virus, most likely from 1969.

Jimmy's doctor explained to him that his liver enzymes were mildly elevated and that he would order the proper test for Hepatic C PCR viral load. This would tell him whether or not Jimmy had the virus now. If he were one of the 15 percent of the lucky ones that get rid of the virus on their own, this test would be negative. Unfortunately, the test came back positive. Given his result, Jimmy's wife had to be tested, too. Luckily, she tested negative for the antibody and had no other prior risk factors. Though it may seem strange, the doctor was not surprised since it is not uncommon to find sexual partners in monogamous relationships (that is, where each partner only has one partner) where the Hepatitis C virus has not been transmitted from one partner to the other—even after a 25-year relationship.

Jimmy was devastated to learn that he had Hepatitis C and concerned about infecting his family, his wife, and his children. Jimmy was encouraged to avoid giving his family members anything that might have come in contact with his blood. For instance, he should not share razors, nail clippers, or toothbrushes with anyone in his family. His doctor reassured him, as well, that the Hepatitis C virus was not acquired through casual contact, such as kissing someone on the cheek, shaking someone's hand, or hugging them, and nothing would need to change in Jimmy's daily home routine.

After getting his test results and talking to his doctors, Jimmy was referred to the liver clinic to evaluate the stage of his disease. There, Jimmy was offered treatment. He had the option of being treated with the FDA-approved, three-times-a-week injection or being enrolled in a clinical trial using a pegylated form of interferon and ribavirin. This new combination medication, he was told, was supposed to have a higher success rate than the three-times-a-week injection, both being offered in combination with ribavirin, a second antiviral medication. Remember, Jimmy is a lawyer. "Clinical trial?" he said. "I do not want to be a guinea pig." The doctor then explained that patients have to be informed of their rights, and have to have every possible side effect of the treatment explained to them *before* the treatment begins. Patients also have the right to refuse at any time to continue participating in any kind of research study.

Because Jimmy will be getting treatment at a health facility where he develops a confidence and trust in his medical team, Jimmy feels comfortable. Jimmy thinks over the possible pros and cons of taking part in the clinical trial. He asks several questions, and is satisfied with the answers. He decides to sign the clinical trial consent form and begins to take a medication that is being studied.

"Theresa": A Puzzle

Theresa is a beautiful 46-year-old bookkeeper in good health. She was sent to the liver clinic in 1999 with a report of abnormal ALT, a liver enzyme. The blood test ordered by the liver specialist, who always looked for the presence of a virus when ALT is elevated, was positive for the Hepatitis C antibody. A second test verified that Theresa was infected. Theresa had never done drugs, never had a blood transfusion, never knowingly had sex with anyone who had Hepatitis C, had no tattoos, and though her ears had been pierced when she was a baby, the pediatrician used a sterile needle. So, after her doctor had questioned her about risk factors, there was still no clue as to the cause of the virus. That remained a mystery, just as it does for about 10 to 15 percent of all cases of Hepatitis C in the United States.

DEALING WITH IT!

Once you have been diagnosed with Hepatitis C, it is important for you to realize that you need to accept it and deal with it—you need to grab the bull by the horns!

Learning to recognize the problem their disease poses and addressing it directly, rather than avoiding it, is one of the lessons infected patients are encouraged to practice as a way of life. While many patients experience a wave of shock or even despair after learning they are infected, usually, once they have understood clearly the diagnosis, many of these same patients will show courage and acceptance.

In most cases, the clinician who informs the patient of the Hepatitis C diagnosis does so with a compassionate and supportive approach. Hopefully, the clinician will also be realistic and informative. It is not easy for *anyone* to inform another that he or she has a serious disease. The clinician should give all the facts and talk about the best, as well as the worst, outcome and express the hope that the disease can be managed. Patients also find courage in the fact that treatment involves teamwork. They themselves must work positively with the medical team that is there to support them by making every effort to minimize possible complications of the disease.

Managing Hepatitis C has been made easier by lessons we have learned in the past 20 years. Patients are less likely to be subjected to guilt and shame, or to feel that their illness is a taboo subject. In that way, we are all far better off than we were in the early 1980s, when the society's attitude toward HIV was too often "You play, you pay."

Because of these social lessons learned, in matters of treatment, we no longer have to invent the wheel. While Hepatitis C is a very different disease then HIV, it is acquired through similar risk factors, and some of the socioeconomic issues are similar. HIV treaters have learned how to encourage people to keep up with their treatments and to make good use of support groups. These leaders have also learned how to involve community churches in raising public awareness and reaching out to people who need help. Now, these lessons are being applied to the treatment of Hepatitis C as well.

CHAPTER FOUR

EVALUATING THE EXTENT OF THE DISEASE

Once you have been diagnosed with Hepatitis C, your medical team will make an evaluation. In some cases the primary-care doctor does the evaluation, but more often the job will be done by a specialist, such as a gastroenterologist or hepatologist, who specializes in liver ailments, or an infectious disease specialist. These specialists are more familiar with the latest treatments for the disease.

Whoever does the evaluation will include the following procedure:

- Document your medical history—that is, take a thorough look at your medical background, lifestyle, and the health history of your extended family
- Give you a physical exam
- Order laboratory testing for Hepatitis C.

Let us look at each of these so you will know what to expect from your doctors.

YOUR MEDICAL HISTORY

Your medical history helps the doctor determine how long you have had the disease. That fact can give an additional clue about how much your liver has been damaged. We know that damage from Hepatitis C progresses slowly over many years, so that if you have had the disease for 20 years, you probably have more liver damage than if you had had it for 10 years. But keep in mind that some livers progress very slowly toward cirrhosis, while others progress quickly.

Your doctor will take a full medical history of your past and present illnesses or medical conditions. He or she will also want to know what medications you are taking now, since some are toxic to the liver and may cause liver enzymes to be elevated. If you have a condition such as high blood pressure or diabetes, the doctor will want to know how well it is being managed. Your doctor will also want to know whether you have had surgery—including oral surgery. In addition, he or she will take a history of any psychological illness you may have had, such as depression or schizophrenia, and want to know how well these conditions are being managed. You will be asked if you had a blood transfusion prior to 1992. Additional questions will explore signs of chronic fatigue, or tiredness, that comes for no apparent reason.

Your doctor will ask (if it applies to you) the following questions:

- Have you been diagnosed with HIV?
- Have you ever had a Cesarean section or other obstetric or gynecological surgery?
- Have you ever had kidney dialysis or been told you have elevated liver enzymes?

The doctor will also ask questions about your lifestyle:

- Have you changed sex partners frequently?
- Have you had unprotected sex?
- Do you have tattoos or body piercings?
- Have you inhaled cocaine?
- Have you injected drugs (even once)?
- How much do you drink, and over how many years?
- Do you smoke, and if so, how much?
- Have you been in the military?
- Have you been in prison?

Do not be offended by these questions. Your answers help the doctor evaluate the extent of your liver disease.

By asking about your family medical history, your doctor can learn whether other family members have Hepatitis C or related medical conditions. That information may point to a source of infection and can sometimes hint at how long you may have had the disease.

Finally, as part of the background information, you will be asked about your job. Some jobs carry special risks of potential Hepatitis C infection. Your doctor, for example, may ask if you have ever come in contact with infected blood, blood products, or needles. Such contact is not confined to hospital workers. It can happen in school clinics and to people who play sports or do physical training. People in law enforcement are at risk of such contact, as are people who work at manual jobs that can cause physical injury. *Any* contact with infected blood carries with it the risk of Hepatitis C.

PHYSICAL EXAMINATION

Knowing what to expect helps you to relax during a medical exam. Be prepared for a detailed exam, and know that such an exam is necessary in order for you to get a careful diagnosis and the very best treatment.

Your doctor will first measure your height and weight, take your blood pressure, and examine your ears, eyes, and mouth. The doctor will do an external examination of your liver by lightly tapping your abdomen on your right side above the liver. The sound the doctor or clinician hears will indicate whether there is an abnormality in the size and/or position of the liver. The healthy liver measures 4–6 inches in height and 6–8 inches in width.

Your doctor will look for certain symptoms:

- Yellowness in the white part of your eyes, which would suggest jaundice
- Dullness on tapping the belly to detect any presence of fluid (a normal belly should not have any loose fluid and should sound hollow)
- Swelling (from accumulation of fluid)
- Spider weblike veins, usually on chest and back
- A large swollen vein around the belly button
- Enlarged breasts in men
- External hemorrhoids.

Lastly, the doctor will take a hand and gently push against the area of the body just above the liver. The normal liver is not tender to the touch.

LABORATORY TESTS

Some of what the doctor needs to know can be revealed only through laboratory tests of your blood. Your doctor will order such tests for your first examination and for all following ones. These diagnostic tests can show if you are infected with the Hepatitis C virus. They can show evidence of the virus even in people who have no present symptoms.

Blood tests can also reveal whether you are infected with HIV and whether antinuclear antibodies (ANA) are present. If they are, that is a sign that the body's own cells are attacking the liver.

A person with Hepatitis C must also be on guard against new infection with Hepatitis A or B because these secondary infections may make the Hepatitis C worse. Through blood tests, your medical team will discover whether you are immune. If you are not, your team will offer vaccines to protect you against Hepatitis A and B. The vaccines are sometimes used singly and sometimes in combinations.

See Appendix A for a list of common blood tests ordered for Hepatitis C.

EVALUATING MEDICAL HISTORY, EXAMINATION, AND TEST RESULTS

After all this diagnostic information has been collected, your doctor will take a close look at your medical history and the results of all the tests. Then he or she can tell you the extent of your disease. After talking with you about your condition and the treatment options, your doctor will give you reading material and, sometimes, videos and Internet addresses. (If you do not have a computer at home, go to your local public library. The librarian there will be glad to help you find the information you need.) Your doctor will also help direct you to information hotlines and support groups of people who have Hepatitis C.

A doctor cannot predict how fast your liver disease will progress, but he or she *can* go over with you the possible complications that may occur over the years, such as cirrhosis or liver cancer. The risk of such complications remains for as long as the infection is present.

The doctor must also decide if you are medically and emotionally stable enough to be a good candidate for treatment with antiviral medications. Such treatment requires a good deal of work from you. For the duration of your treatment, you may have to organize your life around that treatment, making sure that you take *all* your medications *when* you should. In addition, you need to maintain the emotional strength to cope with the symptoms and the treatment. You should be helped by the knowledge that the symptoms will end soon after you complete treatment.

If your doctor believes you have other medical problems in addition to Hepatitis C that need to be addressed, or that at present you are not emotionally ready for treatment, that does not mean you cannot ever receive treatment. It just means he or she will try to bring these physical or emotional problems under control first. Even if you do not take immediate treatment, you still need to be monitored for Hepatitis C at least yearly, with the help of blood tests and an abdominal sonogram. At the end of each year, your doctor can reassess your condition and talk with you again about treatment options.

Whether or not you are in treatment, your doctor will recommend that you avoid alcohol and other substances that may be toxic to the liver. If you take herbal remedies, you will be asked to bring them in and have them checked out so that your doctor can determine if they might be harmful to the liver.

Besides your own well-being, there are others to think about. You certainly do not want to risk infecting other people in your house. You will be advised to avoid transmission of the Hepatitis C virus by not sharing household items, such as razors, toothbrushes, nail clippers, and scissors. You will also be advised that you or your partner should use latex condoms while having sex, unless you have been in a monogamous relationship for over five years and your partner has tested negative for Hepatitis C.

CHAPTER FIVE

TREATMENT OPTIONS AND SIDE EFFECTS

The decision whether to treat or not to treat Hepatitis C is made by two people: you and your doctor.

The doctor's share of the decision is based upon a thorough evaluation of the degree of liver disease and upon the risks and benefits that the patient might receive from treatment. Your decision should be based upon that same information.

Evaluation for Hepatitis C takes several weeks, and that is to your advantage. During the weeks of testing, you have time to review the books, pamphlets, and videos you have been given, and time to write down questions you still need to ask your doctor. Do not be embarrassed about asking questions. Doctors like to work with patients who are well informed and who want to know about their illness—it strengthens the partnership, most likely long-term, between doctor and patient. Until then, your doctor must continue to monitor the disease for possible complications.

If the doctor offers you treatment, you will be the one to make the final decision. Your doctor will offer you treatment only if he or she believes that the risks of treatment, including possible side effects, will be outweighed by the possible benefits of the available treatments.

WHO SHOULD BE OFFERED TREATMENT?

The recent NIH Consensus Conference guidelines state clearly that all patients with Hepatitis C are "potential" candidates for antiviral therapy. However, your doctor must make a reasonable assessment based on your current health, emotional status, and family history. Based on that assessment, he or she may recommend that treatment begin or that it be put off for a while until you are ready to be treated.

WHEN SHOULD TREATMENT START?

While in general it is best to start treatment as early as possible, there are some kinds of situations that might delay treatment:

- If, for instance, the person with Hepatitis C is older, has uncontrolled diabetes, blood sugar in the 350–400 range, and advanced kidney complications, then the doctor must decide if Hepatitis C presents a serious threat compared to these other illnesses. In most cases, the doctor will want to stabilize the patient's diabetes first, then reconsider treatment for Hepatitis C.

- If the person with Hepatitis C is of child-bearing age and wants to have children, the doctor may recommend that she plan to have a child first and then start treatment.
- If the person with Hepatitis C is currently changing jobs or working a double shift, the doctor may suggest that the patient postpone treatment until he or she has a less stressful workload.
- If the family of the person with Hepatitis C has particular needs that take a lot of energy, the patient may want to wait until things are a little less challenging and consider treatment a year later.

Treatment for Hepatitis C may not be an "emergency," but timing may be crucial to the success of the treatment. A year of treatment may be demanding or may go very smoothly—it cannot be predicted. Some people are able to keep up their ordinary lives, but others are not.

WHAT ARE THE TREATMENT OPTIONS?

A doctor selects and recommends a particular medication or combination of medicines because he or she believes that medication has a reasonably good chance of either curing a disease or at least minimizing its effects on the human body. The doctor's selection is based on the results of the medical research approved by the Food and Drug Administration (FDA). By recommending medication, the doctor hopes to improve the quality—and possibly even the length—of the patient's life.

Up until 2002, the most commonly offered treatment for Hepatitis C approved by the FDA was a form of interferon (interferon alfa-2a or interferon alfa-2b). This medication was given three times a week, sometimes in combination with pills of another medication called ribavirin, which is an antiviral drug.

Alfa interferon is a substance our bodies produce naturally in small amounts when our immune system responds to fight infection, or in response to the presence of a foreign body. Alfa interferon is one of many such chemicals that the body produces as part of an immune response. In the face of an attacker as aggressive as Hepatitis C, the body's own immune system may not be enough to overcome the Hepatitis C virus.

THE STANDARD OF CARE

The FDA has approved two forms of interferon. These prescription drugs, in combination with the antiviral pegylated drug called ribavirin, also available by prescription, have become the standard of care in treating HCV. The names of these two combination drug regimens are as follows:

- Pegasys® (peginterferon alfa-2a) with Copegus® (ribavirin, USP) and

- PEG-Intron®* (peginterferon alfa-2b) with Rebetol® (ribavirin, USP).

These forms of interferon are "pegylated," which means that the interferon has been attached to a PEG molecule (polyethylene glycol) that allows it to stay in the blood for roughly a week. The good news for patients is that they can get once-a-week dosing instead of three-times-a-week dosing.

At this writing, these two treatments appear to have similar rates of success in achieving a sustained virological response. But remember, because it is *very* important: success is measured by having no virus detectable for six months after stopping treatment.

Treatment with either combination of medication requires very careful monitoring by a physician. Keep in mind that there is no guarantee of a successful treatment. The success rate of each treatment is measured as the percentage of patients expected to achieve undetected virus levels six months after completing treatment.

At the moment, these treatments appear to be of similar safety and similar efficacy, and it is not within the scope of this book to recommend one treatment regimen over another. That decision will be made between you and your doctor based on the information available at the time of your treatment.

---

* PEG-Intron is a registered trademark of Schering Corporation.

Talk to your doctor about the choice that is best for you. You may bring to the discussion with your doctor whatever information you have gathered from your own reading and consulting. In that way, the final decision becomes a team decision.

BASIC DIFFERENCES IN NEW TREATMENT OPTIONS

We can only outline some of the basic differences between these two new treatments. Check with your doctor to determine how these differences may or may not affect you.

As we mentioned, one of the drugs is called peginterferon alfa-2a (Pegasys), and the other is called peginterferon alfa-2b (PEG-Intron). Both drugs have to be injected under the skin. Pegasys is in liquid form and needs refrigeration. PEG-Intron is in powder form, can be stored at room temperature, and has to be mixed with sterile water prior to injecting.

Ribavirin (Copegus® and Rebetol®) is an antiviral drug. Both Copegus (ribavirin, USP) and Rebetol are taken by mouth with food. For genotype 1, Copegus is dispensed as tablets of 200 milligrams (mg) and prescribed as 1000 mg per day for persons weighing less than 165 pounds. That boils down to five tablets per day taken in two doses. For persons weighing more than 165 pounds, the dosage is 1200 mg per day.

For genotype 2 or 3, Copegus (ribavirin, USP) is dosed

as 800 mg (400 mg in morning and 400 mg in afternoon.) This dose has been found to be sufficient to achieve positive effects.

Pegasys (peginterferon alfa-2a) is given as a fixed dose (180 micrograms) for those of any weight. It is administered as a once-a-week injection under the skin. It is dispensed in a clear liquid in a small glass vial that has to be refrigerated. A member of your medical team will teach you how to draw the liquid with a syringe and how to inject yourself. Treatment is recommended for 48 weeks for genotype 1, a more stubborn strand that requires a longer treatment, and 24 weeks for genotype 2.

PEG-Intron is prescribed according to a person's weight. It is dispensed in four possible vial sizes in the form of a white powder, along with a second vial containing sterile water. Each weekly dose comes with two syringes. One is used to measure the precise amount of water that is added to the vial containing powder. The second syringe is used to draw the newly mixed solution and then inject it under the skin. It does not need refrigeration. Patients are taught how to properly mix the water with the powder.

The FDA has approved a fixed dose of 800 mg Rebetol given as a 400 mg dose twice a day.

One significant study on the use of peginterferon in combination therapy with ribavirin showed significantly lowered response rates among African Americans with Hepatitis C than among Caucasian patients. See

Appendix C for these study results. This was the first study designed to determine the efficacy of this combination treatment specifically for African-American patients. Treatment was successful in 26 percent of cases involving genotype 1, which is the most common among African Americans, and hardest to treat. The study showed that peginterferon alfa-2 in combination with ribavirin was a safe and tolerable treatment for African-American patients with chronic Hepatitis C viral infection.

For patients of all genotypes, the success rate for Pegasys(peginterferon alfa-2a)/Copegus (ribavirin, USP) was 56–61 percent; for PEG-Intron/ribavirin, 54 percent. Genotype 1 high viral load patients represent 50 percent

Figure 7. Efficacy for HCV genotype 1 using peginterferon and ribavirin

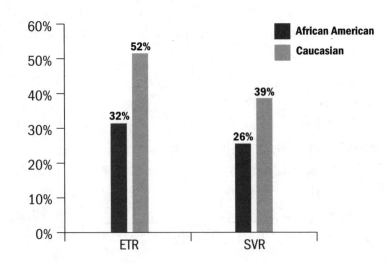

Source: Jeffers, Cassidy, Howell, et al. *Hepatology*, 2002

of the United States' HCV population. What is the significance of high viral load? Approximately two-thirds of all HCV-infected patients have a high viral load, and these patients tend to have lower response rates compared to patients with a low viral load at baseline. Patients with high viral load treated with PEG-Intron/ribavirin achieved sustained viral load rates of 42 percent. Treatment with Pegasys/ribavirin in patients with high viral load resulted in the highest sustained viral load reported in this patient population—59 percent.

The sustained viral load success rate in these patients for Pegasys/ribavirin was 41–46 percent*; for PEG-Intron/ribavirin was 30 percent.[†]

When we look at all infected genotype 1 patients, the success rates using PEG-Intron/ribavirin was 46–51 percent, Pegasys/ribavirin, 42 percent. Clearly there is an urgent need for more clinical trials. At present, we cannot yet explain with certainty why there is an apparently lower success rate among African Americans. But we do know that the slightly lower success rate for African-American patients is *not* due to a lack of compliance. In fact, African Americans were much more compliant than Caucasian patients. Some of the other possibilities that might explain the lower success rates are differences in immune systems or differences in body mass index.

---

* Fried, M. *New England Journal Medicine,* 2002; 347, pages 975–982 and Hadziyannis, S. *Annals of Internal Medicine,* 2004; 140, pages 346–355.

† Manns, M. "Peginterferon alfa-2b plus ribavirin...." *Lancet,* 2001; 358, pages 958–965.

What factors weigh heaviest in terms of outcome, with high viral load being most important? In clinical trials of interferon and peginterferon alfa-2b, genotype and viral load are frequently cited as being the primary drivers of response. Patients infected with genotype 1 have much lower response rates than patients infected with genotypes 2 and 3. There is too little information published at this time on genotypes 4, 5, and 6 to make any valid comments on their response to treatment. Similarly, patients with high viral load tend to have lower response rates than patients with low viral load. Other factors associated with lower response rates include race (African Americans tend to have lower response rates) and whether a patient has advanced liver disease or cirrhosis—as this will also decrease response.*

POSSIBLE SIDE EFFECTS WHILE YOU ARE ON TREATMENT

Treatment for Hepatitis C is no picnic for most people. The side effects are serious. But knowing beforehand what to expect will help you to cope with these side effects. Let us start with the basics:

- No one gets all of the side effects.
- There is no way to predict who will get which ones.

---

* Manns, M. "Peginterferon alfa-2b plus ribavirin. . . ." *Lancet*, 2001; 358, pages 958–965.

- Side effects can last one day, one week, or longer.
- Your doctor has ways to make these side effects more tolerable.

Patients who go into treatment prepared for the worst often find that the treatment is actually easier than they had expected.

Doctors who are not experienced with Hepatitis C treatment are sometimes unwilling to continue treatment after the first few weeks, when the side effects begin. They think that the side effects of the first week or two of treatment will last through the rest of the 48 weeks of treatment, but often this does not prove to be the case.

You will need a doctor and a medical team who are cautious, knowledgeable, and experienced in helping you with the side effects of Hepatitis C treatment. Under such care, the majority of patients tolerate the treatment quite well. Your team, which should include physician assistants and nurse practitioners trained in managing the treatment, will provide ways of dealing with the symptoms. Acting always with your safety as their primary concern, they can help make your treatment a successful one.

THE IMPORTANCE OF COMPLIANCE

While Hepatitis C is very different from HIV, we have learned from HIV patients and from the clinicians who treat them how to manage antiviral treatment in the best possible way to ensure "compliance and adherence." Compliance and adherence describe how well patients follow advice from their doctors and how well they stick to the treatment regimen—that is, taking medications, going for blood tests, and showing up for office visits. In the best cases, patients comply and stick to the doctor's instructions because they understand it is in their best interest.

Why is it important for patients to adhere to the prescribed dose for the duration prescribed? It has been demonstrated that patients with genotype 1 treated with greater than 80 percent of their peginterferon alfa-2b and ribavirin for more than 80 percent of the time and especially in the early part of the treatment, have a higher chance of a sustained virological response* than patients who took less than 80 percent of each drug for less than 80 percent of the time. Therefore, compliance and adherence is critical to ensure the best possible response.

People who do *not* comply often lack information about the seriousness of their illness, about how the medications work, and about how to deal with the side effects of the medications. Report side effects to your doctor when you first experience them, not when they have become intolerable and may be harder to treat. Also, report depression early. Do not let your emotions drive you away from a treatment that can allow you to return to your normal routines and pleasures.

---

* Mchutchinson, John. *Gastroenterology*, October 2003; 125(4), pages 1284–1286.

WHAT YOU NEED TO KNOW

Before a patient starts treatment, he or she is provided an hour-long educational session, scheduled as a visit with the physician assistant or the nurse practitioner. In that session, patients should learn how to take the medications, their possible side effects, and the best ways to keep those side effects under control. Patients are often advised not to depend on their memory, but to write things down. They are also encouraged to bring a family member or friend along to medical visits in order to write down key points.

Women of child-bearing age are warned that ribavirin can cause severe birth defects, and that they can only receive treatment if they have a negative pregnancy test. That test will have to be repeated every month during treatment. We also insist that men and women on treatment use two forms of birth control to avoid pregnancy and continue to do so for six months after treatment ends.

After 12 weeks of treatment, you will be given a blood test to determine your viral load. If the blood test shows a reasonable drop in the virus, continue treatment because now you have a 72 percent chance of success. If the viral load is not significantly reduced, stop treatment because you only have a 2 percent chance of successful treatment.

> *Men and women use two forms of birth control to avoid pregnancy while on treatment and continue to do so for six months after treatment ends.*

During treatment, you will be expected to follow certain instructions:

- Take full doses of both your medications.
- Call your provider with any question or complaint.
- Try never to miss a dose of medication, but if you do miss a dose, never double up on the next dose.
- Inject medication on the same day each week in order to develop a regular pattern.
- Always take pills with food and plenty of liquids.

A special issue occurs because many Hepatitis C patients are between 40 and 60 years old—an age where they need reading glasses. It is essential, of course, not only that you read the instructions given to you, but also that you can tell the difference between the numbers 1 and 2 on the syringe. Your doctor may check your vision and, if needed, refer you to an eye doctor who can prescribe the eyeglasses you need. For many people, the kind of nonprescription reading glasses found in most drug stores will do the trick. Reading glasses also have the benefit of allowing you to read food labels, which helps you to buy the healthiest possible foods when you grocery shop.

WHEN THE GOING GETS TOUGH

Taking Hepatitis C treatment for half a year, or even a year, will get tough at times. While some patients report that they experience no discomfort with it, after three or four months, most patients feel quite tired, and most experience some side effects. Rarely, patients do feel overwhelmed by the treatment and so are given lower doses until the side effects improve. But, of course, it is better to remain at full dose, if possible.

One way to help yourself get through the treatment period comfortably and positively is by joining a support group in your area. In these groups, those with the disease can talk about and share the details of their treatments, side effects, past experiences, and their own ways of dealing with their treatment. Most people going through treatment find such exchanges very helpful. In the description of common side effects that follows, remember that nobody experiences them all and that most patients report that the treatment is easier than they expected.

During the very first two days and possibly the first few weeks following the injection of your medication, you will most likely have some flulike symptoms, such as:

- Sweats
- Headache
- Body aches
- Fatigue.

Of these four, fatigue may be the only one that lasts after the first few weeks. You may feel a little more tired and have less

In the description of common side effects that follows, remember that nobody experiences them all and that most patients report that the treatment is easier than they expected.

energy than usual. If you feel fatigued, try to continue mild activity, such as walking several blocks a day, as long as you are not short of breath. Maintaining a minimal level of exercise has helped many patients keep up their energy. (If you experience shortness of breath or chest pain while walking or exercising, report this immediately to your doctor.)

Some people get headaches. If you experience one, report to your doctor what you are feeling, how long your headache lasts, and what relieves it. Drinking 8 to 10 glasses of water each day may help alleviate headaches and other symptoms. These flulike symptoms can also be controlled by taking acetaminophen or ibuprofen a half-hour before taking your injection—especially the first few times. (Of course, you should discuss this with your doctor.) It is best to inject the medications half an hour before going to sleep so you can sleep off some of the symptoms.

Hepatitis C treatment has sometimes been associated with depression and, in rare cases, suicidal thoughts or suicidal attempts. While not everyone experiences depression when going through treatment, it is a very serious side effect. Before you start treatment, you will be asked if you have ever been depressed and whether you have been treated for depression or any other psychological problem or psychiatric illness. Your health care team may recommend a one-time evaluation by a mental health professional to screen for possible signs of depression that need to be stabilized before you start treatment.

On each visit while you are in treatment, you will be asked to report mood changes. Your spouse, friends, or relatives may be the first to notice such changes. Maybe, with their help, you can identify the situations that make you irritable and find ways to improve them or find ways to cope with those situations better. If your doctor decides that your level of irritability has become a serious issue, he or she may reduce the dosage of your medications for a while. Irritability is a side effect of interferon. In some cases, consultation with a psychologist or other mental health worker may help you manage your irritability.

While you are going through treatment, you may have difficulty sleeping. Warm baths, relaxation techniques, or soothing music often help. Brisk walks outside in the evening may also help you fall asleep. If these methods do not work, your doctor may prescribe a medication that will help you sleep.

Some people experience slight tingling in their fingers when taking medication. If this happens to you, report it to your doctor. The tingling, which may point to a slight irritation to your nervous system, usually goes away after you stop treatment. You and your doctor will decide if this side effect is tolerable for you, or whether you need to take lower doses of medication for a while.

Some people experience a slight loss of taste or a change in how food tastes. Often, you can correct this by using new herbs or spices to season your food. Look for healthy foods that appeal to you and load up on your favorite fresh fruits and vegetables.

You may lose your appetite and not be able to eat large meals. If so, eat small meals more often and eat healthy snacks.

Some people experience nausea. Drinking cranberry juice or ginger ale often helps. So does sucking lemon-flavored lozenges or mints.

A rare but serious side effect of treatment is an increase in liver inflammation and a worsening of liver disease, especially in patients who already have cirrhosis. You will be given periodic blood tests to determine and monitor the level of liver function (PT and albumin).

Your thyroid gland, which is partly responsible for your metabolism, may become underactive or overactive during treatment. Your doctor will be checking your blood every three months to see how well your thyroid functions. This is usually a relatively easy problem to correct with medication that has no serious side effects.

Once a month, or more often, your doctor is going to look for other side effects occurring in your blood cells. You may develop anemia, which means a reduction in your red blood cell count. Red cells are needed to carry oxygen to your brain, your heart, and all your muscles, so your doctor may have to change your dose of medication, or stop it for a while, if you develop anemia. He or she may also choose to give you another medication that will help support your red cells. If your red cells are low, you may feel very tired, and you may even get short of breath when you walk a few blocks. If that happens, tell your doctor right away.

Your white cells also may become low. Because they are needed to fight infection, your doctor will not allow them to drop too low. You need to go for blood tests as often as your doctor tells you—usually once a month, but the doctor may ask you to go more often in order to monitor your blood. If necessary, the doctor will have you lower your dose of medication or will give you medication that stimulates your body to produce more white cells.

Your platelets are cells in your blood that help your blood clot. They may also become lower while on treatment, and they need to be watched.

You will be asked to report any fever or chills and any signs of infection.

Your skin may become dry and itchy. Skin moisturizers will help. Sometimes, if you develop a rash, you may be referred to a dermatologist who may prescribe a lotion that will help.

A slight redness or skin darkening at the spot where you inject medication is normal and sometimes shows up a few days after the injection. It does not usually spread and usually goes away after a few days or a week. It is recommended that you change the area into which you inject every week. For example, you might inject on the inner side of your right thigh during the first week, on the outer side of your right thigh the second week, and the third week, on the inner side of your left thigh. And so on.

You may have some thinning of your hair or some hair loss during treatment. Often, hair loss is insignificant and will correct itself after you have finished treatment.

Avoiding frequent shampoos and using conditioners to moisturize your scalp may help protect you from hair loss.

This long list of side effects should not scare you. They occur in about 10–15 percent of people in treatment. You may experience a few at one time or another. Or you may experience a side effect that has not been reported as often. If you do get a reaction to your medication, tell your doctor immediately. He or she will manage it, keeping your best interests and safety in mind.

Remaining on treatment for the full 24 or 48 weeks of therapy is easier when there is true teamwork between the clinicians and the patient's support team at home. This support team optimally includes your spouse, parents, children, sisters, brothers, and friends. Under the right supervision, 85 percent of patients complete a full course of therapy, unless it is interrupted because of inadequate viral response.

CHAPTER SIX

THE LIVER TRANSPLANT

The medicines available for the treatment of Hepatitis C work for many people. But even when medical treatment fails to keep the liver healthy and functioning, there is still hope. For people with serious liver disease, transplantation is sometimes the only effective treatment. In fact, Hepatitis C is the most common reason people need liver transplants.

Chronic hepatitis and cirrhosis of the liver are diseases that commonly make liver transplantation necessary. Another, rarer disease that can lead to transplantation is inflammation of the bile ducts that lead into the liver.

The purpose of a liver transplant is to replace a diseased liver that can no longer function with a healthy liver. There are two options for liver transplantation:

- Cadaver donor (from a dead or dying person).
  Often livers come from persons who have suffered

brain death as a result of head injury or
hemorrhage.

- Living donor (a healthy person donates part of
  his/her liver). After going through a thorough
  emotional and physical evaluation, a donor will
  spend a week in the hospital after having part of
  his liver removed and will take four to six weeks of
  rest at home.

Eighty to 90 percent of those who undergo a liver
transplantation survive and, after one year, around 80
percent of liver transplants are working well. That number
falls to 60–65 percent after five years. For reasons we do
not know yet, African Americans and Asians do not do as
well with liver transplantation as Latinos or whites. That
means there are more rejections of the transplant and
lower survival rates with African Americans and Asians.

While we await the scientific explanations for the
discrepancy, we can do things for ourselves to improve
those odds. For the patient, it means following the
doctor's instructions scrupulously, both before and after
the surgery. You and your doctor must work as a team to
best assure that you are healthy going into the surgery
and that you get healthy after it is over.

SHORTAGE OF AVAILABLE LIVERS

There is also a role for *all* of us in remedying another part
of the problem. A serious shortage of livers for

transplantation has people waiting in line for an operation that could extend their lives. You will remember that close genetic matching is desirable in transplantations, but too few African Americans are willing to donate organs. The result is that a lot of people are waiting, and sometimes dying, because they cannot get the operation that could give them at least several quality years of life.

We view the shortage of available livers for transplantation as a community problem. Donating organs is an act of great generosity and often gives the blessing of life to someone who might otherwise not receive it. For more information of this subject, the Minority Organ/Tissue Transplant Education Program (MOTTEP) is an excellent resource. The organization is supported by the National Institutes of Health and Howard University. See their Web site: *www.nationalmottep.org/*.

Facing this shortage of livers for transplantation, surgeons are developing new techniques to provide liver tissue for transplantation. For example, a donor liver may be split in half so that it can be transplanted into two recipients. Surgeons have also found effective ways to take liver tissue from a living patient. These new procedures allow a parent's liver to be transplanted to a child; it is also becoming an option for adult recipients.

"TYRELL'S" LIVER TRANSPLANT

Let us take a closer look at liver transplants by following a patient we will call "Tyrell Clark," a resident of Boston.

Tyrell had been carrying Hepatitis C for 30 years before he was diagnosed in the early 1990s. By that time, the disease was in an advanced stage, and Tyrell's own immune system was attacking the bile ducts in his liver. As a result of the attack, bile had built up, damaging the liver cells. In those conditions, liver cancer had developed, and the failure of Tyrell's liver threatened his life.

In 1994 Tyrell had surgery that allowed his bile ducts to flow fairly well. But when the problem returned in 2002, tests showed that his liver tissue was now too scarred to repeat the corrective operation, and he was put on a transplant list. He learned that because the supply of livers was short (only 5,000 of the 15,000 needed) available transplant livers would be given only to those who had the best prospects of a successful graft. Because of Tyrell's poor chances, he was not high on the list. The only alternative for him was a live donation.

Tyrell's brother, Michael, immediately offered himself as donor. Michael and Tyrell did not go into the decision blindly. Both brothers knew of the case at a hospital in New York City in which a donor died as the result of a bacterial infection that resulted from the surgery.

The brothers knew of the risks, even under the best of conditions, but they also knew that at their hospital, all 28 live donors had lived, though about one-third of them had postsurgical complications, such as blood clots, bile leakages, and infections.

Michael was comfortable with his decision to donate part of his liver to his brother. Even to have a chance at lengthening his brother's life made the risks worthwhile. Now Michael was ready to donate 60 percent of his liver, knowing that the liver would grow back, or regenerate, to full size in weeks or, at the most, months.

Once Tyrell and Michael started preparing for the operation, the brothers joked to one another that it seemed as if they were training for a marathon. For months they worked out together—on treadmills, stationary bikes, and in a college swimming pool. It was important that they both be in good health, because this would greatly improve the odds of successful transplant. Mike had also improved the odds by donating two units of his own blood to be used for himself during the surgical procedure if a transfusion was necessary. Now the time had come.

During the operation surgeons discovered that Tyrell's liver was in even worse shape than they had thought. Any further delay would probably have cost Tyrell his life. Instead, two days after the operation, Tyrell was able to leave the intensive care unit. Blood tests showed that his new liver was working.

Michael had poor liver function just after the operation and was jaundiced. But within two weeks his condition improved, and both brothers went home from the hospital.

Even for those patients for whom liver transplant is the only chance at life, needing one does not necessarily mean finding one. The pool of donors is far too small. According to the Westchester County (New York) Medical Center, 954 people in the U.S. died awaiting liver transplants in 1996. The transplant waiting list was nearly four times the number of livers donated. In the past several years, those statistics have not improved much because cases of Hepatitis C and other liver-related problems are on the rise.

DISQUALIFYING RISK FACTORS

You will be disqualified if you have risk factors that mean your chances of long-term survival are slim. The risk factors are as follows:

- Having secondary liver cancer, because this means the cancer has spread elsewhere in the body and a liver transplant is unlikely to check it.
- Having a current or recent drug or alcohol problem. If you have clearly put old bad habits behind you, past drug use should not affect your eligibility for a transplant.
- Certain types of cuts, scars, or complications from previous abdominal surgery. Transplant surgery is complicated and lengthy, and pre-existing scar tissue or adhesions could make such surgery difficult, dangerous, or impossible.
- Being homeless or living in isolation from others may make it difficult to get on the liver transplant waiting list. This is because successful transplantation and good recovery depend on regular physical, emotional, and psychological

support. People who do not have others to help care for them, encourage them, and help them through the emotional rough spots are considered poor prospects for transplantations.

LIVE DONORS: A RARE GROUP OF RISK TAKERS

The fate of many end-stage liver disease patients rests on the kindness of strangers. The better you understand this, the better you will be able to work effectively to get the help you need, to find the patience you need, and to realize what a blessing a donated liver can be.

The first step to understanding is to consider what kind of person would sacrifice part of his or her liver for another person they have never even met. That is a question clinical psychologist Mary Ellen Olbrisch, Ph.D., has been trying to answer. Dr. Olbrisch has been collecting data on this rare group at Johns Hopkins University Medical Center, which has one of the nation's largest living-donor programs for adult liver transplants.

Most liver donor transplants come from people who are biological or emotionally related to the recipient, but a growing number of complete strangers are stepping forward. They are known as Good Samaritan donors.

Why do they give even if it hurts? In a world of givers and takers, these are the givers. Sometimes there is a spiritual component to their generosity. According to Dr. Olbrisch, "All of our donors have a greater willingness to take risks."

When asked how high a risk they are willing to accept in order to donate an organ, given the chance of serious medical complications or death, Good Samaritan donors respond with amazingly high numbers. According to Dr. Olbrisch, "Our data showed that for liver donors, over half were willing to go 75 percent or higher." Meaning they would go forward even if they had a 75 percent chance or greater of experiencing serious medical problems or death.

"When people offer to donate a partial liver to a stranger, the response is usually, 'What's wrong with them?'" Dr. Olbrisch says. But she adds: "I think we need to ask that question, but maybe not as much as people think. Those of us in the transplantation field know it is a very gratifying, exciting thing to do, but a lot of people want to play their part and make a contribution. Donating to a stranger may be no more pathological than wanting to donate to a relative."

CRITERIA FOR TRANSPLANT PATIENTS

Patients must also realize that *both* the recipient and the living donor must meet the specific criteria of each transplant center. Below are the criteria used at one center.

RECIPIENT CRITERIA

- At the present time, living donation will not be offered to patients who have fulminant hepatic failure.

- Recipients must have no evidence of extrahepatic malignancy.
- Recipients must be cleared for transplantation based upon the standard workup.
- Recipients must have no percutaneous stents in place.
- Recipients must have no previous portacaval shunts. (A mesocaval shunt is the only exception.)
- Recipients must have no previous liver resections or biliary reconstruction surgery.

DONOR CRITERIA

- Donors must be 45 years old or younger.
- Donors must have no history of cardiopulmonary, renal, or neurological disease.
- Donors must show no evidence of liver abnormalities.
- Donors must have no previous liver surgery, with the exception of cholecystectomy.
- Donors must have no history of diabetes. Hypertension is permissible if mild and well controlled on medications.
- Donors must have no history of deep vein thrombosis or PE.
- Donors must have no history of bleeding tendencies.
- Donors must be serologically negative for Hepatitis B and C and HIV.

- Donors must have a healthy hepatic vascular system.
- Donors must show no evidence of liver mass.

THE TRANSPLANT EVALUATION

Patients being considered for a liver transplant will meet with members of the transplant team at the center to which they are referred by their doctor:

- The hepatobiliary (liver) surgeon
- The hepatologist (liver specialist)
- The transplant coordinator (nurse, nurse practitioner, or physician's assistant) who will assist in evaluation, education, and postoperative follow-up
- The transplant social worker who will provide support for the patient and the family.

The patient will undergo an extensive evaluation to make sure he or she is emotionally and physically ready for this delicate surgery.

ONCE YOU ARE ON THE LIST

If you are approved for transplantation, you will be placed on the recipient list of the United Network for Organ Sharing (UNOS). Through the network, liver recipients are matched to donors according to blood type, height and weights, the stage of the illness, and the waiting time on the list.

Depending on your medical conditions, you will either wait for your new liver in a hospital or at home. Waiting can be a matter of days or months. During that wait, a clinic or your referring hospital will want to see you regularly to review your condition. Your team recognizes that the waiting period is a difficult time for you and your family. So if you feel unwell or have questions, contact the transplant coordinator, who will be pleased to help you.

When your coordinator calls you on the phone or your pager goes off, contact the hospital's switchboard, give your name, and explain that you are on the liver transplant waiting list and have just been paged by the transplant coordinator. The on-call coordinator will then get in touch with you and let you know what you should do.

You will normally be told to go straight to the hospital. Once you arrive, more blood tests and X rays will be performed, but if a relative or friend has come with you, he or she will be very welcome to stay with you until you go to the operating room. The length of the transplant operation varies but usually takes between 6 and 10 hours on average. If you have had previous surgery, it may take longer.

THE TRANSPLANT PROCESS

The operation itself is long and complex. The surgeon will first peel away the internal organs so that he or she can get to your liver. The blood vessels connected to your liver are then clamped and cut. Blood clotting proteins (normally provided by the liver itself) will be infused into your body, and you will receive a blood transfusion (up to 20 pints) to replace blood that has been lost during the procedure.

During the removal of the liver, a second surgeon will check and prepare the new liver for the transplantation. The replacement liver is then placed in the cavity and stitched (sutured) to the surrounding arteries and veins, and the bile duct of the donor liver sewn to the bile duct of the recipient. The clamps are then taken off. Bile will immediately flow from the new liver. The abdomen will be closed, using special stitches, some of which will dissolve.

Every effort will be made to ensure that you experience as little pain as possible. You will be prescribed pain-killing drugs (analgesics) and will be shown how to take deep breaths and how to move your body in the easiest way.

You will have a large wound in the shape of an inverted T. This will be covered by a dressing.

LIFE AFTER TRANSPLANT

After a liver transplantation, a patient must take a lot of medications to prevent rejection of the new organ. There may be complications, such as a small risk of bleeding, infection, and rejection. The patient will be monitored closely. The medications have side effects, and the team will help to manage them. The success of the surgery will be a result of teamwork with the patient, who is a most important team player. Compliance with the instructions of your doctors will help ensure a good outcome.

It is beyond the scope of this book to address all the issues and questions that arise when someone needs a liver transplantation. All transplant centers have specialized in addressing all issues concerning the individual who needs a transplant. In this book, it is our goal to make you aware of the real but remote possibility that exists for anyone who has Hepatitis C that their liver may one day be unable to function and they may indeed in the future need a new liver.

A common question of liver transplant patients is, "How long will it be before I am 'out of the woods'?" After the first month, the risk of organ rejection decreases, and so too does the level of antirejection drugs the patient must take. Six months after the transplantation, the patient's dose will be reduced even further.

Another more grave question the patient will typically ask is, "How long can I expect to live?" This is difficult to predict, but the odds look pretty favorable and continue to improve. More than 90 percent of people with transplants survive for at least one year, and around 65 percent survive for at least five years.

CHAPTER SEVEN

CO-INFECTION OF HEPATITIS C WITH HIV

Co-infection is the term used to describe the condition of patients infected with more than one virus. In most cases, it refers to people who have human immunodeficiency virus (HIV)/acquired immunodeficiency syndrome (AIDS) *and* Hepatitis C virus (HCV), although the term is also applied to patients with Hepatitis C and either Hepatitis A or Hepatitis B. Nevertheless, the most serious combination is HCV and HIV/AIDS.

For a person who has HIV, it might seem that the worst nightmare would be to find out that one also has Hepatitis C—another serious disease! But that is not always the case. If you spend enough time in an HIV clinic, you will come to know the kind of individuals that struggle with a life-threatening illness, how they think and how they survive. Most of these people are brave fighters. According to most of them, the worst already happened when they initially found out they had HIV. Once they come to grips with that reality, nothing else could shake them. They were involved with a strong support system, whether through the HIV clinic, special services, or a hospital with a strong focus on HIV. Having HIV in the new millennium is associated with a life-saving support system: all issues that challenge the HIV-infected person are addressed from medical to social to nutritional to psychological to financial. Whenever a problem arises, there is a team that can address that problem.

Of course, we are referring to those HIV persons who have accessed the services available to them. We are not in any way minimizing the seriousness of having both HIV and HCV. It is indeed a real health hazard. But at least we in American live in a time when HIV treatment has reached a point where HIV-infected people can have their disease stabilized and can benefit from being almost assured of a normal life span with protection from most HIV complications. It is not the gloomy picture that existed 20 years ago or that exists today in other parts of the world. As a matter of fact, at least 40 percent of all HIV persons have HCV. This is not surprising considering both illnesses share many of the same risk factors.

Either of the two infections (HIV and HCV) represents a serious challenge for the patient. But put them together and a whole new set of variables enters the equation, and recovery is drastically complicated. The two viral infections, with their unusual characteristics and treatment requirements, may work against each other.

Worse yet, HIV accelerates the progression of HCV-related liver disease—the most grueling consequence of Hepatitis C. The problem also works the other way; HCV may also affect the course and management of HIV infection. One serious outcome is that people who are co-infected develop severe liver damage, such as cirrhosis, at a much higher rate than those who do not.

Let us make clear that having HIV is not "the same" as having HCV. The differences:

- HCV is more common among IV drug injectors and is more easily transmitted than HIV. With HCV, a high viral load does not mean you will get sicker faster.
- HIV is less common in IV drug injectors and less easily transmitted than HCV. With HIV, a high viral load is associated with getting sicker faster.

If you have both HIV and HCV, your liver disease will progress faster to cirrhosis, and you are more at risk for complications of liver disease, such as liver cancer. The cruel reality is that you may be less likely to get a donated liver if you should ever need transplantation.

HOW SERIOUS IS THE PROBLEM OF CO-INFECTION?

Extremely serious. Consider that in the U.S. alone, 40 percent of those who tested positive for HIV are also afflicted with HCV. The number exceeds 400,000 people.

The likelihood of co-infection is dramatically higher among men and women who contracted HIV by bloodborne virus than in those infected as a result of sexual intercourse. That case is made in dramatic fashion by the following statistics:

- The co-infection rate is just over 50 percent for patients who acquired HIV by using a contaminated apparatus for intravenous drug injection.
- That rate rises to 70 percent for hemophiliacs who acquired HIV through contaminated transfusions of blood.
- The prevalence of HCV is less than 3–5 percent for persons infected with HIV by sexual intercourse, as long as they have no history of either transfusions or IV drug use.

The Centers for Disease Control (CDC) points out that because Hepatitis C is primarily transmitted among IV drug users, co-infection is common in this group.

Also, co-infection is almost as common among those with hemophilia who received clotting factor concentrates (blood products that help hemophiliac patients prevent bleeding).

TREATMENT OF CO-INFECTION

A few years ago, HIV patients had little hope when the disease progressed from HIV to AIDS. The end result was that patients were severely limited in their function, if they were able to function at all. Because there were not treatments that resulted in improvement or even relief, most HIV-infected individuals just waited to die.

Things have changed!

At the cutting edge of the change are highly active antiviral therapies (HAART) anchored by drugs that come in two classes—reverse transcriptase inhibitors and protease inhibitors. This treatment dramatically alters the course of HIV infection. Today, most HIV patients are prescribed a combination of three or four of these drugs, and most patients experience significant improvement.

From 1995 to 1997, the percentage of AIDS patients treated with HAART increased from less than 10 percent to over 80 percent. The rate of hospitalization fell from 6.4 days to 1.1 outpatient days a year. HAART also brought a dramatic decrease in the incidence of the major "opportunistic" infections: pneumocystis, pneumonia, mycobacterium avium complex disease, and cytomegalovirus retinitis. After HAART was introduced, death from these diseases dropped from 15 percent to less than 2 percent.

Sometimes it is difficult to know why some individuals with HIV and HCV are less responsive to treatment. Is it the co-infection or is it deeper than that? For instance, many men and women who are co-infected have conditions or factors such as major depression or active alcohol or drug addiction that prevents or complicates the effectiveness of antiviral therapy.

People with chronic Hepatitis C who continue to abuse alcohol are at risk of ongoing liver injury. Furthermore, their antiviral therapy may not work. Strict abstinence from liquor is required during therapy, and interferon should be given with caution to a patient who only recently stopped drinking. Usually, a six-month period of being alcohol free is required before starting therapy on such patients.

The same period of being "clean" is recommended for IV drug users before starting therapy. When patients have a history of abuse, any therapy should be accompanied by treatment for the continuous substance abuse.

Because of the obvious complexities, treatment for co-infected patients should be done by health care providers with considerable experience treating such people or those with experience conducting clinical trials. How can you find out about the qualifications of your doctor? Ask! Check out their information. Be sure! Talk to your local librarian about how to determine a doctor's credentials and qualifications. Whether you are a patient or have a loved one who needs to know, finding the best doctor is an important step to recovery.

CO-INFECTION AND THE THREAT TO THE LIVER

Co-infected patients may have a greater risk of developing hepatocellular carcinoma, the medical name for a certain form of liver cancer. In the past, people with co-infections were not even considered for liver transplants. Doctors believed that because people who had received liver transplants would have to take immunosuppressive drugs for a lifetime, the treatment would devastate the already weakened immune system of HIV-positive individuals.

Since then, tests show that the use of immuno-suppressive drugs may actually thwart the progression of HIV because it prevents the replication of the virus. That virus reproduces by integrating into the DNA of T-lymphocyte immune cells. As immunosuppressive drugs restrain the production of immune cells, they also prevent the HIV from reproduction fast enough to take advantage.

PREVENTION OF CO-INFECTION

As with most illnesses, the best cure is prevention. Those living with HIV who are not already co-infected with HCV can take measures to dramatically reduce the odds of acquiring the Hepatitis C virus. At the same time, taking these steps will also reduce the chances of transmitting AIDS to others.

The first and most significant step to preventing the spread is to stop doing what is most responsible for it. Not injecting or stopping injection drug use would eliminate the chief source of infection. For the addict, this likely requires substance-abuse treatment. We strongly recommend relapse-prevention programs.

Those who continue to inject should at least receive counseling about safer injection practices. That means using new, sterile syringes every time they inject drugs. It also means never reusing or sharing syringes, needles, water, or drug preparation equipment.

Those who do not use drugs also need to take precautions. They should never share toothbrushes, razors, or other personal-care items that might be contaminated with blood. Though the CDC says data is incomplete, tattooing and body piercing may be a source for infection with bloodborne pathogens and should be avoided.

Is safe sex a preventative for HCV and AIDS co-infection? Not all the data is in, so it is better to be safe than sorry. Practice safe sex and avoid multiple sex partners. In those ways you can avoid infecting others.

It is also critical that co-infected individuals avoid drinking alcohol in excessive amounts. The best advice is not to drink at all if you are already fighting HIV and HCV because even moderate to small amounts of alcohol can have a bad effect on the liver. Damage can be done with the consumption of as little as one 12-ounce can of beer a day, one 5-ounce goblet of wine, or one 1.5-ounce shot of hard liquor.

Because of the possible harmful effects of certain medications on the liver, even those medications bought over the counter should be used only after consulting with a physician. The same precautions should be taken with the use of alternative or herbal medicines, according to the CDC.

Individuals infected with both HIV and HCV should be vaccinated for Hepatitis A as well as Hepatitis B. The CDC says that the vaccines appear safe for these patients, and more than two-thirds of those vaccinated develop antibody responses.

There is no question that co-infected people must live carefully and take full advantage of the best treatments available. That means taking the best possible care of themselves, taking the medications their doctors prescribe, as directed, and always showing up for scheduled checkups.

Many people are doing just that—being strong in their determination to live.

CHAPTER EIGHT

YOU ARE NOT ALONE: FAMILY AND SUPPORT GROUPS

Hepatitis C is too heavy a burden to bear alone. You need practical and emotional help from others. How do you find it? Well, the first move is yours; be honest with yourself and with the people who matter most. Tell others about the diagnosis and let them know, when they ask, how you are doing as you battle Hepatitis C. Such openness is a way of using your personal support system. Some people may offer you help, such as a ride to the clinic or a prepared meal when you are not up to preparing one yourself. Others will just listen, and that can be of great value to you emotionally.

Some people are open to everyone and, in this way, enjoy the advantage of a broad support group. Others settle for a small select circle of loved ones and friends.

Opening up, even to near and dear ones, is not always easy. There is a stigma attached to Hepatitis C, similar to that attached to HIV/AIDS. However, it should be stressed that Hepatitis C is not HIV and does not carry the identical burden. Too many people try to hide their conditions from others. The result is that these people come to think of the disease as a dirty secret. Such a stance can prevent diagnosis and treatment. It can also injure the spirit, just when the infected person most needs a strong spirit.

We have come a long way since the discovery of HIV/AIDS in dealing with the stigma of that disease. The world has learned to approach illness with compassion, without judging its morality. People infected with HIV have come to accept their diagnosis with courage and determination and to avoid people who choose to stigmatize and look down on them because they have a serious illness that is associated with a high-risk lifestyle. If you have such an illness, pay no attention to those who might judge you.

As many as 15–20 percent of those who have Hepatitis C have no idea how they were infected! Should they be targeted with accusations of high-risk behavior? Should anyone ever be targeted? Or rather should the community direct its emotional energy at viewing all persons infected with a virus as innocent victims of life's hazards?

For example, take Andrew, who is now 36 years old. He showed up in our clinic for the first time six months ago. As usual we took a detailed history to assess the extent of his liver disease. He had joined a rehab group six months earlier and had been drug and alcohol free for six months. Andrew was eight years old when he had his first heroin injection, and nine years old when he started drinking a fifth of rum per day.

At the rehab center, he had been told that he had Hepatitis C and did not have any other disease. We explained to him the need to do further testing. We advised him to have a liver biopsy to determine the extent of damage to his liver. He responded by telling us that he was going to do everything we suggested to get his health in order and to avoid the complications of liver disease. Andrew stated very calmly and clearly that these last six months were the first time in his life that he could remember being sober and they were the first time he slept under a roof that was his own, bought his own groceries, and put them in his own pantry. He was determined not to wreck this chance at a normal life.

For Andrew, growing up in the streets meant committing any crime in order to survive. He somehow managed to avoid spending time in lockup. But he did not know how to read or write, and he had learned how to count only from fellow addicts. Now he was taking a literacy class.

He had also found God. In short, this man, who became a drug addict at eight years old, had turned his life around. Who would judge him and stigmatize him? The Bible holds that only God is the true Judge. In medicine, the same policy is taught: never pass judgment regardless of anyone's behavior or criminal or moral history. No one knows what circumstances have led people to risky behaviors.

When it comes to your disease, you may or may not know how it was acquired. And you learn the value of compassion. You come to appreciate the discretion of your friends in not questioning you, and you suffer from the indiscretion of those who pry for details. Out of fear of disclosure, people may avoid getting tested, or if they *do* get tested, they may conceal the outcome from others. That means that these people are not only hurting themselves psychologically but also that they risk passing the disease on to the people who are closest and dearest to them.

Project "Be Hepatitis C SMART" (an acronym for Shattering Myths and Reinforcing Truths), under the sponsorship of the American Gastroenterological Association (AGA), has launched a national campaign to educate the public, health care providers, and Congress about prevention, diagnosis, and treatment of Hepatitis C. AGA also conducted an online survey of 1,226 people from the general population who were not infected with HCV, which included 493 infected individuals and 415 physicians (198 primary-care physicians and 217 specialists).

The survey found that, while Hepatitis C does carry some stigma, patients themselves, out of paranoia, often think the situation is worse than it really is. Patients believe that others associate Hepatitis C with drug addiction and unhealthy lifestyles; but it turns out that, in fact, only 30 percent of those interviewed harbor such beliefs.

Yes, some people *do* believe Hepatitis C patients have lived promiscuous, loose lives. Some even associate the disease with sin and moral decay. But the plain fact is that Hepatitis C infection has been reported as a result of accidents among health care providers, contact with injured soldiers in Vietnam, hemophilia, blood transfusions, getting tattoos and body piercings, and several other causes.

Yes, people are entitled to their beliefs. But when those beliefs harm others, maybe we need to re-examine them. Doctors see the sad results of secrecy every day in their offices. When it is time to ask where the patient may have gotten the infection, a surprising number say they just do not know. Too often, it turns out, the patient doesn't know because he or she was infected by another person, who wholly out of shame, failed to give any warning.

We can take an important step toward containing the epidemic simply by remembering that Hepatitis C is a disease, not a curse from God. In the face of disease, the task is to comfort and heal. Not to judge. It is bad enough to be diagnosed with Hepatitis C without being made to feel guilty and isolated.

Ironically, Hepatitis C is significantly undertreated, even among infected white upper-middle-class persons. The reason might well be that, out of fear of stigmatization, people hide their infections, sometimes even from themselves. Doctors will tell you that even people who have clearly been diagnosed are not always willing to do something about it. While they might be walking around carefree, in 20 years some of them will be buried, and the others will be waiting for liver transplants.

With so much widespread ignorance on the topic of Hepatitis C, the process of revealing the problem to others is complicated. Nonetheless, it is an issue that must be dealt with by every Hepatitis C patient.

WHO DO I TELL, AND WHEN AND HOW?

Certainly, you are not going to want to tell everyone about your disease, but there are people you *must* tell. Among others, this means people you might have infected, such as

- People who might have shared your toothbrush, razor, or manicure scissors
- People with whom you have shared an IV drug needle.

If you use IV drugs, to continue the practice of needle sharing is irresponsible. It greatly decreases your chances for recovery and survival, and it spreads the epidemic to others. If you insist on continuing to inject, at least tell anyone with whom you share needles that you are infected.

You should also share your diagnosis with your spouse or sexual partners. The risk of sexual transmission is less than 1 percent, but there *is* a chance, and you owe it to others to warn and protect them.

Some people think that Hepatitis C can be spread by hugging or kissing, but that cannot happen unless, somehow in the process, contaminated blood from one partner is passed to the open-mouth sore or bleeding gums of another. There must be blood-to-blood contact from transmission. The rate of sexual transmission is, in fact, less than 1 percent.

In any case, if you have been diagnosed HCV-positive, it is a good idea for your long-term partner or spouse to be tested. And both of you should recognize that even if the results return positive, it does not mean one individual necessarily "caught it" from the other.

Even if it strongly appears that one person infected the other, it is wasted energy to point fingers. Keep in mind that because Hepatitis C is a new disease, a lot of people experience the symptoms long before they finally get diagnosed. Whether to tell children depends largely on their age and ability to understand what you are saying. But what you *do* need to do is make it impossible for children to access your razor, toothbrush, or any of the other items that may be contaminated.

Whether to tell your parents is another decision each individual must make. No matter how frequently it happens, most people cannot get accustomed to the fact that children may die before their parents. And despite the most optimistic outlook, Hepatitis C is life threatening.

While the decision about who you tell is one you must make for yourself, keep in mind that none of us benefits from bottling our pain up inside or pretending that it is less hurtful—physically and psychologically—than it is. Many doctors are convinced of the health benefits of a positive attitude and strong support system. Such supports actually seem to help your body fight the disease, whether it be Hepatitis C or other serious ailments.

FINDING PEOPLE WHO CARE

In a perfect world, Hepatitis C virus patients could find all the love, support, and understanding they need among relatives, friends, and co-workers. Unfortunately, some people in those groups may be more of the problem than the solution in your quest to recover good health. Maybe they just do not give you anything to cling to, and you still feel isolated and, because you are alone, somehow guilty as well. You may find the resources in Appendix D helpful in getting information and support for Hepatitis C.

Some people find support through activism. They become advocates for research and public information on Hepatitis C, co-infection, or liver disease. If you want to go that route, you can volunteer for a local liver or hepatitis organization, or start a letter-writing campaign to lobby state and federal legislators to make this issue a priority. Some people diagnosed with Hepatitis C organize or participate in walkathons, help put together benefit fundraisers, and find many other ways to make sure people have the right kinds of information. The more people there are who understand, the quicker we will control the epidemic. And you may be surprised by the energy you draw from this kind of activism—energy you need as you face the challenges of your personal fight with the disease.

One organization reaching out is called HCV Anonymous. It is a program of Positive Attitudes Anonymous, aimed at people who have a potentially terminal illness. It helps organize groups that help one another in this new way of life. Here, people keep each other's confidences, in their pursuit of what members want today and in the future.

Members of HCV Anonymous reach out to individuals like themselves, who are dejected and depressed because of their condition, and who no longer live life to its fullest. Members reach out to those who have become disoriented and lead them to some peace of mind. People who attend HCV Anonymous meetings regularly and work in their programs begin to feel more upbeat and are ready to face a potentially terminal illness with a positive attitude and sense of resolve.

HCV Anonymous is just one of the many resources you will discover once you begin to explore what is available to you (*www.hcvanonymous.com*). For the many other resources, see Appendix D: Resources.

BLOOD TESTS

There are a number of common blood tests involved with diagnosing Hepatitis C that your doctor may recommend you have. Among them are the following:

- *Hepatitis B surface antibody.* If the results are positive, this test reflects immunity. If the test results are negative, the patient should receive a set of three vaccines—one now, another one month later, and one in six months.
- *Hepatitis B core antibody.* If results are positive, this test reflects prior infection and immunity, in which case the patient does not need vaccine.
- *Hepatitis A IgG.* If negative, the patient needs a vaccine against this virus—one now and one in six months.
- *Liver biochemical/function.* These tests measure various enzymes released by the liver into the

blood, and also measure other liver functions. Liver enzymes may be elevated when damage occurs in the liver.

- *Complete blood counts (CBC)* measure the three components of blood: red cells, white cells, and platelets.
- *Red cell count* reflects the body's ability to carry oxygen to cells, and also measures the size of red blood cells. The most important red cell count values are *hemoglobin and hematocrit* (together referred to as H&H), which measure the blood's ability to provide the body with oxygen. A low H and H indicates anemia, a serious condition that produces fatigue. Advanced liver disease can produce anemia.
- *White cell count* provides information on the body's ability to fight infection. A high total white count means the body is actively fighting; a low total white count means that the body's ability to fight infection is weakened. Low white blood count may be caused by advanced HCV disease or by HCV medications.
- *Platelet count* provides information on the blood's ability to clot. Low platelet count (thrombocytopenia) is dangerous because of the risk of internal and external bleeding. (Normal platelet count range is 150–350 K/cmm.) Advanced liver disease and HCV medications can cause thrombocytopenia.

- *Chemistry panels* measure minerals (electrolytes), sugar (glucose), and fats (lipids) in the blood, and also measure liver and kidney functions. Lab reports tell your doctor whether liver and kidney functions are normal.

- *Antibody tests* detect the presence of antibodies to the Hepatitis C virus, such as ELISA and RIBA.

- *The ALT test* measures levels of alanine aminotransferase (ALT), an enzyme produced in the liver cells. High ALT levels can be a sign of Hepatitis C, but other conditions can also cause an increase in ALTs. These conditions include heart attacks, high triglyceride levels, and other forms of hepatitis. Many people with Hepatitis C have fluctuating or normal ALT levels, so a normal ALT test does not necessarily mean that Hepatitis C infection can be ruled out.

- *Liver biopsy* involves collecting a small sample of tissue the size of half a matchstick from your liver by passing a needle through the skin into the liver. The sample is then examined under a microscope. Before taking the sample, the doctor applies a local anesthesia to numb the area where the needle will be. Your doctor may ask you to hold your breath for a second or two while this is done. An ultrasound scan may be used to guide the needle. You will need to stay under observation for several hours after the biopsy, but most people return home the same day.

- *Liver/abdominal CT scan* is a form of X ray that
  creates an image of the inside of the body. The
  scanner's computer analyzes the data to build a
  view of the tissues and organs of the body. Almost
  any part of the body can be scanned.

You will be given detailed instructions about preparing
for the scan when you make your appointment. The scan
is likely to involve an injection of contrast dye, in which
case you will be asked to fast for two or more hours. (Take
your regular medication as normal.) You may also be
required to drink a few cups of a special mixture to make
your bowel visible on the scans. The contrast dye is
injected into the vein to make certain regions of the liver
more visible.

This test requires that you lie on the scanner bed and
keep very still. The table will slowly move in and out of the
circular opening of the scanner. You may be instructed to
hold your breath for a short period of time. A specialized
imaging technologist performs the scan. He or she will
see and hear you at all times and assist you if needed.

- *Liver/abdominal ultrasound* uses sound waves, not X
  rays, to generate images. A probe, called a
  transducer, is passed over the skin. The transducer
  sends out sound waves that pass through the body
  and are echoed back. These echoes are transmitted
  to a computer, which interprets the echo data as
  pictures of internal organs and tissues.

This test is used to monitor for the size of the liver, to examine the gall bladder, and to look for bile duct dilatation, gallstones, and any masses that could be signs of developing cancer.

- *Genotyping.* If you do test positive for Hepatitis C, your doctor or the specialist to whom you have been referred will probably order a genotyping blood test. The Hepatitis C virus has at least six distinct forms, or genotypes, labeled 1 through 6. In the United States, about 70 percent of patients have HCV genotype 1. In other parts of the world, other genotypes are more common. Genotype 1 is associated with a poorer response to treatment. Genotyping can help your doctor determine the appropriate Hepatitis C treatment and how long treatment should be given.
- *HCV RNA tests.* Unlike antibody tests, HCV RNA tests directly measure for the presence of the Hepatitis C virus. HCV RNA tests may be qualitative or quantitative.

  - *Qualitative HCV RNA tests* are used to diagnose Hepatitis C. Your doctor might choose to perform an HCV RNA test instead of the ELISA, especially if you are at high risk for Hepatitis C. The HCV RNA test gets results in as little as one to two weeks after exposure. A positive HCV RNA test means a person has Hepatitis C infection.

– *Quantitative HCV RNA tests* allow your doctor to
determine exactly how much viral load you have.
A higher viral load is not always a sign of more
advanced disease, but it can indicate how well
the patient will respond to treatment. These tests
are also used to monitor response to treatment.
For example, if the viral load decreases during
treatment, this suggests that treatment is working
and should be continued. If the viral load
remains the same, the patient is not responding
to treatment.

- *Alpha-fetoprotein tests.* Alpha-interferon is a marker
of liver cancer, and a mild elevation in alpha
fetoprotein is sometimes seen in Hepatitis C. It is
an alarm signal if your alpha fetoprotein
progressively goes up during treatment. This test is
needed every 6 to 12 months to monitor for liver
cancer in patients who have cirrhosis.

- *Bilirubin test.* Bilirubin is a yellow pigment that
becomes elevated when red blood cells are not
properly excreted by the liver. The test is used to
screen for and monitor liver disorders, such as
jaundice, or liver diseases, such as cirrhosis. It is
done if your doctor thinks you have symptoms of
liver damage or liver disease. In adults, a blood
sample is taken from a vein in the arm; in newborns,
a blood sample is taken from the baby's heel.

- *Albumin test.* Albumin is a protein synthesized by
the liver that circulates in the blood. Low albumin

levels indicate poor liver function and contribute to the accumulation of fluid in the feet and ankles. It is sometimes seen in very late stage liver disease. Albumin levels are usually normal in chronic liver disease in the early stages. Normal range is 3.5–5.3 g/dl.

- *Prothrombin time (PT)* is a blood clotting test given when the blood concentrations of some of the blood clotting factors made by the liver are low. In chronic liver disease, the PT is usually not elevated until cirrhosis is present and liver damage is fairly significant. Normal range is 10.4–12.9 seconds.

- *Thyroid function tests.* If treatment is being considered, this test provides a baseline. Treatment with interferon may cause the thyroid gland to become overactive or underactive.

APPENDIX B

FREQUENTLY ASKED QUESTIONS ABOUT VIRAL HEPATITIS C

What are the specific blood tests you can have to check for Hepatitis C? There is more than one test available to see if you have been infected with Hepatitis C. Your doctor may want to do just one or a combination of them. They are as follows:

- *EIA or Enzyme Immunoassay.* This is usually the first test done. If positive, your doctor should confirm the results with the laboratory.
- *RIBA or Recombinant Immunoblot Assay.* A supplementary test.
- *Anti-HCV.* This test will not determine if you have chronic (long-term) or acute (recently infected) Hepatitis C.
- *PCR or Polymerase Chain Reaction.* This test is available commercially. PCR determines the presence of the Hepatitis C virus.

Can you have a "false-positive" test result? Yes! You will find this more in people with a very low risk of HCV, such as blood donors. If your test comes back positive, another test should always be done to insure it is not a question of "false-positive" results.

What is the next step if your results are positive? If your test results have been confirmed as positive, make an appointment with a physician specializing in Hepatitis C.

Can Hepatitis C be spread during medical or dental procedures? There is no evidence that HCV can be spread in most doctors' or dentists' offices in the United States. But hemodialysis patients are at increased risk of getting Hepatitis C.

Who should get tested for Hepatitis C?
- Persons who ever injected illegal drugs, including those who injected once or a few times many years ago
- Persons who were treated for clotting problems with a blood product made before 1987 when more advanced methods for manufacturing the products were developed
- Persons who were notified that they received blood from a donor who later tested positive for Hepatitis C
- Persons who received a blood transfusion or solid organ transplant before July 1992 when better testing of blood donors became available

- Long-term hemodialysis patients
- Persons who have signs or symptoms of liver disease (e.g., abnormal liver enzyme tests)
- Health care workers after exposures (e.g., needle sticks or splashes to the eye) to HCV-positive blood on the job
- Children born to HCV-positive women

What is the next step if you have a confirmed positive anti-HCV test? Measure the level of ALT (alanine aminotransferase, a liver enzyme) in the blood. An elevated ALT indicates inflammation of the liver, and you should be checked further for chronic (long-term) liver disease and possible treatment. The evaluation should be done by a health care professional familiar with chronic Hepatitis C.

Can you have a normal liver enzyme (e.g., ALT) level and still have chronic Hepatitis C? Yes. It is common for persons with chronic Hepatitis C to have a liver enzyme level that goes up and down, with periodic returns to normal or near normal. Some persons have a liver enzyme level that is normal for over a year, but they still have chronic liver disease. If the liver enzyme level is normal, persons should have their enzyme level rechecked several times over a 6- to 12-month period. If the liver enzyme level remains normal, your doctor may check it less frequently, such as once a year.

TRANSMISSION

How can a person have gotten Hepatitis C? HCV is spread primarily by direct contact with human blood. For example, you may have gotten infected HCV if you:

- Ever injected street drugs, as the needles and/or other drug utensils used to prepare or inject the drug(s) may have had someone else's HCV-infected blood on them
- Received blood, blood products, or solid organs from a donor whose blood contained HCV
- Were ever on long-term kidney dialysis, as you may have unknowingly shared supplies/equipment that had someone else's infected blood on them
- Were ever a health care worker and had frequent contact with blood on the job, especially accidental needle sticks
- Have a mother who had Hepatitis C at the time she gave birth to you, during which time the infected blood may have gotten into your body
- Ever had sex with a person infected with HCV
- Lived with someone who was infected with HCV and shared items such as razors or toothbrushes that might have had his/her blood on them.

Can Hepatitis C be spread by sexual activity? Hepatitis C is not very often spread by sexual activity. However, you should always use condoms and take precautions against sexually transmitted diseases, such as AIDS, Hepatitis B, gonorrhea, or chlamydia.

Can HCV be spread by oral sex? There is no evidence that HCV has been spread by oral sex. See the section on counseling for more information on Hepatitis C and sexual activity.

Can HCV be spread within a household? Yes, but this does not occur very often. If HCV is spread within a household, it is most likely due to direct exposure to the blood of an infected household member.

Since more advanced tests have been developed for use in blood banks, what is the chance now that a person can get HCV infection from transfused blood or blood products? Very little chance. The tests in use today are sophisticated enough to almost always detect Hepatitis C.

PREGNANCY AND BREAST-FEEDING

If you are pregnant, should you be routinely tested? Testing for Hepatitis B and C is now routine for pregnant women. If you are a woman who could be pregnant and you have Hepatitis C, you must take a pregnancy test before, during, and for six months after treatment ends to make sure you are not pregnant. During treatment, and for six months after treatment, female and male patients must:

- Use two forms of birth control (one being a condom with spermicide)
- Tell your doctor right away if you or your partner becomes pregnant.

What is the risk of spreading HCV to your newborn infant?
Approximately 5 percent of infants born to HCV-infected
women become infected. This occurs at birth and no
treatment can prevent it from happening.

Should a woman with Hepatitis C be advised against breast-feeding? Breast-feeding rarely results in HCV transmission.
The U.S. Public Health Service does not advise against it.

COUNSELING

How can persons infected with HCV prevent spreading HCV to others?

- Do not donate blood, body organs, other tissue, or semen.
- Do not share personal items that might have your blood on them, such as toothbrushes, dental appliances, nail-grooming equipment, or razors.
- Cover your cuts and skin sores to keep from spreading HCV.

How can people protect themselves from getting Hepatitis C and other diseases spread by contact with human blood?

- Do not ever "shoot" drugs. If you shoot drugs, stop and get into a treatment program. If you cannot stop, never reuse or share syringes, water, or drug utensils, and get vaccinated against Hepatitis A and Hepatitis B.

- Do not share toothbrushes, razors, or other personal-care articles. They might have blood on them.
- If you are a health care worker, always follow routine barrier precautions and safely handle needles and other sharp instruments. Get vaccinated against Hepatitis B.
- Consider the health risks if you are thinking about getting a tattoo or body piercing. You can get infected if
  - the tools that are used have someone else's blood on them or
  - the artist or piercer does not follow good health practices, such as washing hands and using disposable gloves.

What can you do to protect your liver if you have Hepatitis C? To keep damage and inflammation at bay, the following actions are advised:

- Stop drinking alcohol.
- See your doctor regularly.
- Do not start any new medications or use over-the-counter herbal and other medicines without your doctor's knowledge.
- Get vaccinated against Hepatitis A and B.

What other information should patients with Hepatitis C be aware of?

- HCV is not spread by sneezing, hugging, coughing, food or water, sharing eating utensils or drinking glasses, or casual contact.
- Persons should not be excluded from work, school, play, childcare, or other settings on the basis of their HCV infection status.
- Involvement with a support group may help patients cope with Hepatitis C.

What are the chances of people with HCV infection developing chronic liver disease, cirrhosis, liver cancer, or dying? Of every 100 people infected with HCV, approximately:

- 85 may develop chronic Hepatitis C disease.
- 15 may develop cirrhosis over a period of 20 to 30 years.
- One to five may die from long-term complications (e.g., cirrhosis) or liver cancer.

What is the treatment for chronic Hepatitis C? Of antiviral drugs, such as interferon alone or in combination with ribavirin, are approved for treatment. Interferon works in 10 to 20 persons out of 100 treated. When interferon is combined with ribavirin, USP, the numbers go up to 30 to 40 persons out of 100. Ribavirin alone does not work.

Should persons with chronic Hepatitis C be vaccinated against Hepatitis B? If persons are in risk groups for whom Hepatitis B vaccine is recommended, they should be vaccinated.

What are some side effects of interferon therapy? Most people get flulike symptoms—such as chills, fever, headache, muscle and joint aches, and rapid heartbeat—early on, but they decrease in intensity over time. Later side effects may include fatigue, hair loss, low blood count, depression, moodiness, and an inability to concentrate. Severe side effects are rare.

What are some side effects of ribavirin therapy? Ribavirin can be extremely harmful and cause birth defects in an unborn baby. Female patients and the female partners of male patients should avoid getting pregnant. Ribavirin is known to cause anemia (low red blood cells), which can make heart disease worse. Patients and their health care providers should carefully review the manufacturer's production information prior to treatment for more information and warnings.

GENOTYPE

What does the term genotype mean? Genotype refers to the genetic makeup of an organism or a virus. There are at least six distinct HCV genotypes identified. Genotype 1 is the most common genotype seen in the United States.

Is it necessary to do genotyping when managing a person with chronic Hepatitis C? Yes, as there are six known genotypes and more than 50 subtypes of HCV, and genotype information is helpful in defining the epidemiology of Hepatitis C. · Knowing the genotype or serotype (genotype-specific antibodies) of HCV is helpful in making recommendations and counseling regarding therapy. Patients with genotypes 2 and 3 are almost three times more likely than patients with genotype 1 to respond to therapy with alpha interferon or the combination of alpha interferon and ribavirin. Furthermore, when using combination therapy, the recommended duration of treatment depends on the genotype. For patients with genotypes 2 and 3, a 24-week course of combination treatment is adequate, whereas for patients with genotype 1, a 48-week course is recommended. For these reasons, testing for HCV genotype is often clinically helpful. Once the genotype is identified, it need not be tested again; genotypes do not change during the course of infection.

Why do most persons remain infected? Persons infected with HCV mount an antibody response to parts of the virus, but changes in the virus during infection result in changes that are not recognized by pre-existing antibodies. This appears to be how the virus establishes and maintains long-lasting infection.

Can persons become infected with different genotypes? Yes. Because of the ineffective immune response described above, prior infection does not protect against re-infection with the same or different genotypes of the virus. For the same reason, there is no effective pre- or postexposure prophylaxis (i.e., immune globulin) available.

HEPATITIS C AND HEALTH CARE WORKERS

What is the risk for HCV infection from a needle-stick exposure to HCV contaminated blood? After needle-stick or "sharps" exposure to HCV-positive blood, about 2 (1.8 percent) health care workers out of 100 will get infected with HCV (range 0 percent to 10 percent).

What are the recommendations for follow-up of health care workers after exposure to HCV- positive blood? Antiviral agents (e.g., interferon) or immune globulin should not be used for postexposure prophylaxis. For the source, baseline testing for anti-HCV is recommended. For the person exposed to an HCV-positive source, baseline and follow-up testing is recommended, including:

- Baseline testing for anti-HCV and ALT activity.
- Follow-up testing for anti-HCV (e.g., at four to six months) and ALT activity. (If earlier diagnosis of HCV infection is desired, testing for HCV RNA may be performed at four to six weeks.)
- It is also recommended that there be confirmation by supplemental anti-HCV testing of all anti-HCV

results reported as positive by enzyme
immunoassay.

Should HCV-infected health care workers be restricted in their work? No. There are no recommendations to restrict a health care worker who is infected with HCV. The risk of transmission from an infected health care worker to a patient appears to be very low. As recommended for all health care workers, those who are HCV-positive should follow strict aseptic technique and standard precautions, including appropriate use of hand washing, protective barriers, and care in the use and disposal of needles and other sharp instruments.

APPENDIX C

STUDY ON THE USE OF PEGINTERFERON

Peginterferon Alfa-2a (40KD) (Pegasys®) and ribavirin, USP, for Black American patients with chronic Hepatitis C genotype 1.

Lennix J. Jeffers, Miami VA Medical Center, Miami, FL; William Cassidy, Louisiana State University Health Sciences Center, Baton Rouge, LA; Charles D. Howell, University of Maryland School of Medicine, Baltimore, MD; K. Rajender Reddy, University of Pennsylvania, Philadelphia, PA; Susan Sheridan, Irwin Ho, Sarkis Khouri and George Harb, Roche Laboratories Inc., Nutley, NJ.

Background: Response rates to interferon (IFN) therapy appear to be lower in African-American (AA) patients with chronic Hepatitis C than in Caucasians (Ca). The lower response has been attributed, in part, to the high prevalence of infection with Hepatitis C virus (HCV) genotype 1 among the AA population. However, low numbers of AA patients in prospective clinical trials has hampered meaningful evaluation of antiviral therapy.

Objective: To determine the efficacy and safety of peginterferon alfa-2a (40KD) in combination with ribavirin, USP (RBV) in non-Hispanic AA HCV genotype 1 patients. The trial enrolled patients in a 3:1 ratio of AA to Ca patients and was powered only to estimate sustained virologic response (SVR) in the AA group to within ± 10 percent of 95 percent confidence interval.

Methods: Patients with previously untreated chronic HCV genotype 1 and elevated ALT received peginterferon alfa-2a (40KD) 180 µg sc once weekly plus RBV 1000 or 2300 mg orally based on body weight (<75 kg or >75 kg) for 48 weeks, with 24 weeks of treatment-free follow-up. High viral load (HVL) was defined as HCV RNA >1 X 106 IU/mL. Early virologic response (EVR) at 12 weeks of therapy (defined as HCV RNA <50 IU/mL, or >2-log10 drop in HCV RNA from baseline) was assessed. SVR was defined as undetectable HCV RNA at week 72; sustained biochemical response (SBR) was defined as normal serum ALT at week 72. Histologic responses were reported as Knodell HAI scores of liver biopsies obtained prior to treatment and within 4 weeks of completion of the 24-week untreated follow-up period.

Results: A total of 106 patients received at least one dose of study medication. Baseline characteristics of AA patients were: mean age 46 years, 56 male (72 percent), meal ALT 63 U/L, high viral load 45 (58 percent). Baseline characteristics of Ca patients were: mean age 45 years, 17 male (61 percent), mean ALT 64 U/L, high viral load 12 (43 percent). Sixty-two of 78 (80 percent) AA patients and 22 of 28 (79 percent) Ca patients completed treatment. The table on the following pages shows an SVR rate of 26 percent for AA patients and 39 percent for Ca patients. A larger proportion, 45 of 78 AA patients had high viral loads prior to the initiation of therapy, contrasting with only 12 of 28 Ca patients. SVR was achieved by 9 (20 percent) and 3 (25 percent) of patients with HVL in each group respectively. Of 47 AA patients who had EVRs, 20 patients went on to achieve an SVR. The negative predictive value of EVR was 100 percent for both AAs and Cas. SBR was observed with similar frequency for both racial groups (36 percent for AA and 39 percent for Ca). Histologic analyses of a subgroup of patients for whom paired biopsies were available showed that 13 of 53 (25 percent) AA patients and 1 of 16 (6 percent) Ca patients had fibrosis improvement. No unexpected adverse events (AEs) occurred during the study. Four of 78 (5 percent) AA patients and 4 of 28 (14 patients) Ca patients withdrew prematurely for AEs or laboratory abnormalities.

Conclusions: The SVR of 25 percent in AA with genotype 1 HCV after therapy with peginterferon alfa-2a (40KD) plus RBV is the highest response to combination therapy yet reported in this population. The SVR rate in the AA population is nonetheless lower than in other studies with patients of diverse ethnic backgrounds and may be explained by the higher viral titers observed in these patients. Failure to achieve EVR has a high negative predictive value for SVR with continuing therapy. This study demonstrates that peginterferon alfa-2a (40 KD) in combination with RBV is a safe and tolerable treatment for AA patients with chronic HCV genotype 1 infection. In addition, the SVR rate and histologic benefit observed in this trial provide a basis for future efforts to increase efficacy in this difficult to treat population.

Summary of Efficacy Analyses

Response Variable	African Americans (n=78)	Caucasians (n=28)
Sustained virological response (SVR) Number (percent)	20 (26 percent)	11 (39 percent)
95 percent CI for percentage with response	16–35 percent	21–57 percent
Sustained biochemical response (SBR) Number (percent)	28 (36 percent)	11 (39 percent)
95 percent CI for percentage with response	25–26 percent	21–57 percent

Commercial Relationship: L.J. Jeffers, Hoffmann-La Roche I; W. Cassidy, Hoffmann-La Roche I; C. Howell, Hoffmann-La Roche I; K. Reddy, Hoffmann-La Roche I; S. Sheridan, Roche Laboratories Inc. E; I. Ho, Roche Laboratories Inc. E; S. Khouri, Roche Laboratories Inc. E; G. Harb, Roche Laboratories Inc. E.

Category: JO3 HCV: Clinical Trials and Therapeutic Developments

Keyword: Clinical trials; Ethnic-racial groups; Hepatitis C; Hepatitis C, therapy

Parallel Session 10, Hot Clinical Topics in Hepatology—Sunday October 26, 5:45-6:00 p.m.

Source: Jeffers LJ, Cassidy W, Howell CD, et al. Peginterferon alpha-2a (40kd) and ribavirin for black American patients with chronic hepatitis C genotype 1. *Hepatology.* 2004;39: 1702-8.

Louisiana State University Health Sciences Center; University of Maryland School of Medicine; University of Pennsylvania; Roche Laboratories, Inc., Nutley, NJ.

APPENDIX D

RESOURCES

We have emphasized in this book how important it is for you to get credible information and, where appropriate, to pass it on to others. The available sources for information are countless, thanks to the Internet. A random check of one server revealed more than half a million sites.

In an effort to keep you from having to start from scratch, here are a handful of references that will help you get started:

American Liver Foundation
75 Maiden Lane, Suite 603
New York, NY 10038
800-GO-Liver (800-465-4837) or 888-4HEP-USA (888-443-7872) or
212-668-1000
212-483-8179 (fax)
info@liverfoundation.org

Hepatitis Foundation International
504 Blick Drive
Silver Spring, MD 20904-2901
800-891-0707 or 301-622-4200
301-622-4702 (fax)
hfi@comcast.net

Hepatitis Association of Delaware
100 West 10th Street #409
Wilmington, DE 19801
302-421-3677
302-421-3678 (fax)
www.hadinc.org

PUBLICATIONS AVAILABLE ON THE WEB

Centers for Disease Control and Prevention. Recommendations for Prevention and Control of Hepatitis C Virus (HCV) Infection and HCV-Related Chronic Disease. MMWR 1998;47(No. RR-19):1-39. Available at: *ftp.cdc.gov/pub/Publications/mmwr/rr/rr4719.pdf*

Centers for Disease Control and Prevention. 1999 USPHS/IDSA Guidelines for the Prevention of Opportunistic Infections in Persons Infected With Human Immunodeficiency Virus: U.S. Public Health Service (USPHS) and Infectious Diseases Society of America (IDSA). MMWR 1999;48(No. RR-10):32-34. Available at: *www.cdc.gov/mmwr/preview/mmwrhtml/rr-4810a1.htm*

ADDITIONAL INTERNET RESOURCES

MedlinePlus
www.nim.nih.gov/medlineplus/hepatitisc.html

Centers for Disease Control and Prevention (CDC), Division of HIV/AIDS Prevention
www.cdc.gov/hiv

CDC, Division of Viral Hepatitis
www.cdc.gov/hepatitis

National Institutes of Health
www.niddk.nih.gov/health/digest/pubs/chrnhepc/chrnhepc.htm

CDC National Prevention Information Network
www.cdcnpin.org

For more information on participating in clinical trials for Hepatitis C, visit *www.clinicaltrials.gov*

INDEX

African Americans and
    Hepatitis C, 15, 18, 19,
    33–36
  IV drug users and, 34
  why so few get diagnosed,
    16, 33–34, 37
AIDS. *See* HIV and
    Hepatitis C
albumin test, 98, 140–141
alcohol. *See also* cirrhosis
  alcoholic hepatitis, 22, 48,
    49, 52
  and co-infections, 122
  and Hepatitis C, 52–53
  and liver, 47–48, 49–52
alpha-fetoprotein tests, 140
ALT (alanine
    aminotranserase) test,
    26, 137, 145, 153

American Liver
    Foundation, 161
antibody tests, 23, 26, 135,
    137, 143, 145, 153–154
antiretroviral drugs, 83–90,
    150–151, 155–158. *See
    also* interferon
  HAART for co-infection,
    119
  reducing side effects of,
    151

Banks, Dr. Alpha, 33
bilirubin test, 26, 140
biopsy, 7, 137
blood tests, 77–78, 135–141,
    143–144, 153–154
  false-positive, 144
  for viral load, 93